T0248019

FuelUp

FuelUp

HARNESS THE POWER OF YOUR BLENDER AND "CHEAT" YOUR WAY TO GOOD HEALTH

**DANA COHEN, MD
AND COLIN SAPIRE**

HAY HOUSE LLC
Carlsbad, California • New York City
London • Sydney • New Delhi

Copyright © 2024 by Colin Sapire and Dana G. Cohen
Published in the United States by: Hay House LLC: www.hayhouse.com®
Published in Australia by: Hay House Australia Publishing Pty Ltd:
www.hayhouse.com.au
Published in the United Kingdom by: Hay House UK Ltd: www.hayhouse.co.uk
Published in India by: Hay House Publishers (India) Pvt Ltd: www.hayhouse.co.in

Indexer: J S Editorial, LLC
Cover and Interior design: Julie Davison
Interior photos: Images used under license from Shutterstock.com

Cataloging-in-Publication Data is on file at the Library of Congress

Hardcover ISBN: 978-1-4019-7734-4
E-book ISBN: 978-1-4019-7735-1
Audiobook ISBN: 978-1-4019-7736-8

10 9 8 7 6 5 4 3 2 1
1st edition, September 2024

Printed in the United States of America

This product uses responsibly sourced papers and/or recycled materials.
For more information, see www.hayhouse.com.

Dr. Dana

For my husband, Henry

—————————————

Colin

For my family

Contents

Quick-Start Guide

Establishing and sticking to healthy eating habits can be hard, so we are starting you off with two Fuel Up Habits that are good for you, easy to do, and can make a real difference in how you feel—all at the same time! They are the kind of simple things that will help you "cheat" your way to good health.

Even if you read no further (though we certainly hope you will!), you can start feeling the benefits of *fueling up* right away by doing these two things:

1. **Start Your Day with Water:** Drink a large glass of water when you wake up in the mornings, maybe with a squeeze of lemon juice and/or a pinch of salt (we'll explain why in the book). Do this before you consume anything else.

2. **Enjoy a Smoothie with Benefits for Breakfast:** Designed as delicious and satisfying meals in themselves, our Smoothie with Benefits recipes are packed with a wide variety of nutrients and include protein, a healthy fat, and a generous dose of fiber—all things you need to start your day feeling energized and fully fueled. Recipes begin on page 173, and there are plenty to choose from, so pick one that tantalizes your taste buds!

Healthy Eating Shouldn't Be So Hard

Healthy eating was always a challenge for Colin. He describes himself as a "supertaster"—someone with a heightened sense of taste—which, for him, meant he grew up despising the taste of vegetables. This was particularly true of the bitter ones that are supposed to be so good for you. Broccoli, spinach, cauliflower—they all turned his stomach. Instead, his tastes ran more toward burgers and fries. He could plop down on the couch to watch television and polish off a whole box of cookies in one go, but a green salad . . . not a chance.

As Colin grew older, his need for better nutrition grew more important. His career as an entrepreneur was often hectic and demanding, and he found that he needed regular exercise to keep up with it all. To this day, if he doesn't sweat in the mornings, he just doesn't feel like he has the energy, outlook, or confidence he needs to be productive. He's also a longtime runner, and by the time he reached his 40s, he had found that burgers and cookies were no longer cutting it to fuel his runs. He began choking down a small salad before his usual dinner to provide at least some of the nutrients he'd been missing, but it

1

just didn't feel like enough. It didn't feel practical or sustainable either, because he *really* didn't like that salad.

This was a big part of what motivated Colin to develop the hugely popular NutriBullet® blender and, more recently, the Beast® blender, which launched in 2021. These were more than just business ventures for him. They were also ways to make the healthy foods he had been avoiding more palatable and easier to consume in larger quantities.

Colin knew that to live the life he wanted to live and to feel the way he wanted to feel, he needed better fuel. He needed to find ways to consume all the healthy foods that would help him feel energized and alert on a daily basis and that would help to stave off illness and disease in the long run.

Colin started by making smoothies in his blender and sneaking in those less tasty but nutrient-rich ingredients with ones he enjoyed. Dates have always been a favorite, and they obscure the flavor of most greens. He experimented and found that foods like apples, citrus, and nut butters also did the trick. He now has a veggie-packed smoothie every morning, and that's in addition to *enjoying* (key to making this sustainable) other nutrient-rich blended recipes throughout the day, like soups, marinades for meat, and even desserts. He calls it "cheating"—his way of quickly, easily, and deliciously *upleveling* the nutrition in his meals so he gets all the high-quality fuel he needs to be at his best.

It has been a sustainable cheat too. He has been eating like this for 15 years, and along the way, something interesting happened. He has become something of a veggie convert. He consumes, and even kind of likes(!), a greater variety of vegetables, the kind that used to turn his stomach. He even started an edible garden in his backyard that he picks from each morning for his blends. He still has a burger and fries sometimes, but that's just one part of an overall healthy eating pattern that works for him. Now in his 60s, he has never felt better in his life!

Why We Need to Cheat

People often use the word *cheat* as a way of admonishing themselves or expressing guilt about the foods they have chosen. *I was bad today—I cheated on my diet by having a donut.* Or, *Today is my cheat day, when I get to eat the things I actually like!*

We think that's a pretty disempowering way of thinking about food, so we would like to redefine the concept of "cheating" when it comes to what you eat. Instead of making you feel bad, we would like to turn it into a strategy that you can actually embrace. For us, a "cheat" is any tool or strategy that makes it easier, more satisfying, tastier, or more sustainable to eat healthier. That's because we all know that we should be eating healthy foods, but just because we know something doesn't mean it's easy to do.

Colin's quest for better fuel led him to consider whether he was hydrating well enough to keep up with his active lifestyle and whether his blender could help. He met Dr. Dana when he contacted her about a book she had co-authored on the subject. Blending can be a great tool for staying hydrated, of course, but Dr. Dana was equally interested in how Colin was using it to uplevel his nutrition.

As an integrative physician, Dr. Dana spends a lot of time talking with patients about what they eat, and she has witnessed the profound difference that healthier habits can make in their lives. She has also seen how confusing media messages and the persistent influence of diet culture have failed people. Early in her career, she worked for the famed Dr. Atkins, the first to popularize a high-protein, low-carb way of eating, and she saw firsthand how his and similar methods just don't work long term. Too often the focus is on weight loss over health (they are *not* one and the same), and the weight people do lose rarely stays off for long. In fact, these kinds of diets often lead to unhealthy patterns of gaining and losing, gaining and losing, which obscures the true goal of healthy eating—which is to give our bodies the fuel they need to function well and feel good! What she really wanted for her patients—and for herself!—was to find ways to help her patients eat better that actually worked for them. And not just for the duration of a diet, but over the course of their entire lives.

Of course, that goal can be challenging for so many of us. As a culture we have a complicated relationship with food. We have so much: visit most grocery stores, and you will find a dizzying array of options from around the globe—so many, in fact, that it can be mind-boggling to figure out what to buy. We consume so much—to the point where, as we all know by now, a majority of Americans are classified as overweight or obese. And yet, despite all this abundance, most of us are actually undernourished.

You read that right. We still have widespread nutritional deficits in our culture. Consuming more and having more food options has simply not led to better nourishment, or *fuel*, in much of the Western world. Consider that:

- Just 10 percent of Americans eat enough vegetables to fully fuel themselves.[1]
- Just 12 percent of Americans eat enough fruit to get all the nutrients they need.[2]
- Just 1 in 20 Americans get the amount of fiber their bodies require.[3]

These statistics are pretty surprising when you think about it. We have so much in this country, and yet practically no one is getting everything they need from their food. And these kinds of deficits have real consequences. Our bodies are amazing machines. All on their own, they can ward off pathogens, clear toxins from our systems, heal our wounds, power us through our days, and more, but they need a continual supply of nutrients to perform these remarkable feats.

For example, magnesium—which can be found in a wide variety of plant foods like seeds, nuts, grains, and leafy greens—is crucial for energy production and plays a key role in how our bodies handle stress—and yet, magnesium shortfalls are not uncommon.[4] Another example is fiber, which is present in many fruits, whole grains, and legumes. It feeds our microbiome, which, as we are becoming increasingly aware, is linked to both our physical and our mental health—and yet hardly anyone gets enough of it.

We could provide a hundred such examples. When left unchecked, being undernourished and underfueled leads to an increased risk of a host of chronic conditions, including diabetes and cardiovascular disease. There is evidence that nutrient deficits are contributing to the skyrocketing number of autoimmune diseases and nondescript and formal gut issues being diagnosed in so many people today.[5] Research suggests that eating the recommended amounts of fruits and vegetables is associated with a reduced risk of everything from migraines to infections to eczema and more.[6] It has even been estimated that one in five deaths across the globe is attributable to a less-than-optimal diet—more than any other risk factor, including tobacco.[7]

But this is about more than just disease prevention. It's also about how you feel on a daily basis, which is surely not at your best if you are chronically underfueled. There is even some evidence to suggest that a healthy diet is linked to happiness![8,9,10] More research is needed on that front, but we do know that poor-quality fuel can result in fatigue, brain fog, lousy sleep, diminished immunity, and so much more that essentially amounts to a diminished quality of life.

Like a car running on fumes, when people are underfueled, they simply don't have what they need to run the way they are meant to. And it really doesn't have to be that way.

Your Blender as Delivery System for Good Health

The problem is clear, and we believe that blending is the solution—that it can be the ultimate tool for "cheating" your way to good health!

For most of us, changing our diet is the fastest way to improve our health because it empowers us to provide our remarkable bodies with the fuel they need to do their jobs. We know we should be eating better. (It was the top New Year's resolution for 2022.[11]) We know there are risks if we don't. We know that many of us walk around feeling less than our best too much of the time, and we know that we want to feel better. But all that falls firmly into the category of *easier said than done.*

Here's why the humble blender can make a real difference: we believe your blender is the easiest, most effective, and most accessible delivery system for the nutrients your body needs to perform at its best. If you know how to use it strategically, your blender can be a fast track to good health. That's because blending has some built-in health benefits, including:

Increasing Nutrient Volume: Federal recommendations say that adults need at least 1½ to 2 cups of fruit and 2 to 3 cups of vegetables each day.[12] They also say that most adults need between 22 to 34 grams of fiber each day[13] (though Dr. Dana believes it should be even more than that). All that is a challenge for most of us to consume, but when broken down and concentrated in a smoothie, sauce, or condiment, it's much easier to meet your daily requirements—which is what you need, not only for your overall health, but also to reduce cravings since you are less likely to reach for unhealthy stuff when you feel full and nourished. Blending also makes it easier to sneak in those healthy ingredients that you or your kids may not like. Despite its much-touted benefits, a lot of people don't really like kale, for example, but blend it with apple for sweetness or pineapple for tartness, and it suddenly becomes more than palatable. It becomes something people actually take pleasure in consuming—and pleasure is key to sustainable habits.

Increasing Nutrient Variety: Blending not only allows us to get *more* good stuff into our diets; it also allows us to get a *greater variety* of good stuff. As we all know, different foods provide different nutrients, and in fact, new research suggests that consuming 30 different kinds of plants each week can have real health benefits.[14] Blending makes it more likely that you will get all the many different micronutrients (vitamins and minerals) and phytonutrients (plant-based nutrients) you need to fully fuel your body. It can be a pain to make a couple different vegetable sides for your rotisserie chicken, for example, but it's not at all difficult to throw 3, 5, 7, even 17 different plants into a blender and hit blend. To make a sauce. A soup. A dip. A smoothie. By using your blender, you can layer on different plants, getting a greater variety of different nutrients in the process. The blending recipes in this book will provide you with options for getting the full spectrum of nutrients that your body wants and needs.

Enhancing Nutrient Absorption: Just because we swallow the nutrients we need doesn't always mean that our bodies fully absorb them. This is the problem with many supplements, for example—they can go right through us! There's evidence to suggest that blending might increase the bioavailability of food by breaking it down into smaller particles, thereby allowing you to absorb more of the nutrients inside.[15] There's even some evidence that the act of "wounding" plant foods prior to consumption—through cutting, grating, or use of a blender blade—may release beneficial compounds.[16] More research is needed to draw any firm conclusion on these topics, but what we do know is that digestion begins in the mouth, when you chew up your food to break it down. The problem is that we live in a grab-gulp-swallow-and-go culture, so often forgetting to fully chew our food, which can be taxing on the digestive system. Blending can compensate for a lack of chewing, breaking up particles so they can be more easily digested. We're not going to ask you to blend all your food, of course, but blending some of it may help with nutrient absorption.

Better Hydration: Getting and staying hydrated may be the best way to cheat your way to good health. From proper digestion to immune function, our bodies need to be well hydrated to work properly. Plus, it's another great way to keep cravings in check. Did you know that the symptoms we read as hunger are often really a result of being thirsty? And yet, so many of us are not well hydrated, and the old adage of drinking eight glasses is nothing more than myth. Blending works better. Fruits and veggies, herbs and greens—these things are made mostly of water, so you can help meet your hydration requirements by releasing the water already in plants through blending. Our collection of recipes for what we call Enhanced Water Infusions and Hydration Blends provide additional and, we believe, better hydration options that taste great too!

Fast-and-Easy Healthy Meals: A blender is not an air fryer or an Instant Pot. You don't need a manual to learn how to use it or hours to wait before something is ready to eat. In fact, a blender doesn't take a lot of time or effort at all. You can simply throw ingredients in without measuring (a great cheat) and make recipes like smoothies that don't involve cooking at all (another cheat!) in order to create healthy, well-balanced meals that taste great too. It's a versatile tool that busy people can work into their lives without a lot of fuss. Plus, it's cost-effective. Most people already have a blender in their kitchens, and for those who don't, it's a relatively inexpensive addition. Sure, there are a lot of high-end versions on the market these days, which have their advantages. We are Beast users ourselves, of course, but the strategies and recipes in this book will work with any blender.

The Fuel Up Approach

We want you to eat well because of the many benefits it can bring to your health and well-being. But, to accomplish that easier-said-than-done goal, we understand that people need healthy eating strategies that are accessible, appealing, and even fun—otherwise, they are simply being set up to fail, like so many diets have done to them for so many years.

As we mentioned, Dr. Dana has seen many, many people fail and worse, yo-yo up and down over the years on various diets, which leaves them feeling hopeless, disempowered, and even shameful about being unable to stick with something without cheating (in the traditional sense of the word). And she knows what that feels like. She had her own experience with feeling like a failure when she was a young doctor who smoked a pack of cigarettes a day. She was so ashamed of her habit that she hid it from her colleagues. She was a doctor, after all, so she knew how detrimental smoking could be to someone's health, but she had been doing it since she was a teenager and she just didn't feel like she could stop.

Dr. Dana tried and failed and tried and failed to kick the habit, until she finally went to a psychologist who specialized in a treatment approach called "harm reduction." The psychologist suggested that she stop beating herself up about smoking and, instead, start from a place of acceptance and even radical love for *all* of herself, including the part of her that wanted a cigarette. That meant no more self-shaming when she had one. "If you lived in Paris, where it's much more socially acceptable to smoke, your self-esteem wouldn't be so tied to your habit," her psychologist pointed out. "In fact, if you're going to have an after-dinner cigarette, you might as well enjoy it." This was a paradigm-shifting way of thinking for Dr. Dana, one that completely changed both her mindset and her behavior. She no longer felt bad about smoking, and that freedom allowed her to focus more on what she wanted, which was ultimately to give it up for health reasons. Amazingly, two weeks later, she was able to quit cold turkey. And once she quit, she never went back. She still considers it one of her greatest accomplishments!

Harm reduction is a form of psychotherapy that has been developed to treat substance abuse and addiction. "The essence of harm reduction is the recognition that treatment must start from the client's needs and personal goals," wrote Andrew Tatarsky, author of a textbook on the subject, "and that all change that reduces the harms associated with substance use can be regarded as valuable."[17] It has been described as a philosophy based in "compassionate pragmatism,"[18] which means that when you take a harm-reduction approach, any steps in the right direction are celebrated, no matter how small. And any steps in the other direction are accepted, not judged as bad or wrong. There is no cheating in the negative sense of the word. Shame and beating yourself up simply have no practical or compassionate purpose.

The approach is referred to as "harm reduction" when it comes to addressing substance abuse and addiction. When it comes to food choices, we like to call it being a "good-enough eater." In our view, health*ier* is always a choice worth feeling good about, even if it's not what some may consider the "perfect" choice. That's because, over time, those healthier choices can add up and have a real impact.

This means that if eating several cups' worth of fruit and veggies every day sounds like a lot, then just aim for *more* than what you are eating right now. Even just a little more can be "good enough." And then, maybe somewhere down the line, after you have had a chance to experience how much better healthier eating makes you feel, you will be motivated to step things up even further.

This means that if you want something a little less healthy for dinner, like Colin's former favorite, the burger and fries, maybe you will consider pairing it with something healthy like a side vegetable or one of our nutrient-rich condiment recipes so you can uplevel the nutrition in your meal and still find pleasure and satisfaction in what you're eating.

It also means that if it's your birthday and you like birthday cake, then you should eat the cake. We don't call that cheating. We call that living. (Congrats on being another year older, by the way.)

We know that healthy eating isn't always easy, but it's a whole lot eas*ier* if you don't feel like you have to be perfect or make the so-called right choice every time you want something to eat. We want you to feel good about what you eat. And we want what you eat to make your body feel good—healthy, energized, empowered, satisfied, and happy.

In short, we want you to enjoy what you eat, no matter what choices you make. That's important for a lot of reasons. It's important because your happiness, your sense of well-being, and the pleasure you get out of life is important. It's also important because when researchers looked at what makes a positive difference in someone's eating habits, they found that focusing on the "pleasure of eating" can be key.[19] If you enjoy what you eat, if you enjoy the process of fueling yourself, you are more likely to make healthy choices, not less healthy ones. And not for nothing, but blending, in addition to all the benefits already mentioned, can be a lot of fun for the whole family. And fun habits are that much harder to break.

The Fuel Up Approach

- Start by accepting where you are and build from there.

- There are no food choices that mean you are "bad," have done something "wrong," or are truly a cheater.

- Any improvement is to be celebrated. Progress = success!

How to Use This Book

We aim to make the healthy-eating advice in this book as simple, straightforward, and accessible as possible so that making real and sustainable changes to the way you eat is as easy as possible. We want this to be the kind of book you *use,* rather than just read. With that in mind, each of the main chapters is built around a core Fuel Up habit that, with the help of your blender, will provide you with better fuel to protect your health and power you through your day. Those habits include:

Fuel Up Habit #1: Kick off your days with a blended meal from our Smoothies with Benefits Program.

Fuel Up Habit #2: Start shifting the balance in your eating pattern to favor more natural (and often yummier!) options and fewer ultra-processed foods (UPFs).

Fuel Up Habit #3: Eat more kinds, more colors, and just more plants!

Fuel Up Habit #4: Be more intentional about getting and staying hydrated, because your life literally depends on it!

Fuel Up Habit #5: Make healthy eating more sustainable by getting creative with your food.

We offer brief explanations of the science behind the advice we offer, but the primary goal is to help make this simple, straightforward advice doable for real people with real lives and real tastes for different kinds of foods. Dr. Dana sees this as one of her primary roles as a physician: to make the wealth of information on good health and healthy eating both accessible and actionable. One of Colin's primary motivations for creating his blenders has been to make healthy eating more practical and enjoyable too. These are the same aims that we have for this book.

If you are short on time, or are simply not much of a reader, our most actionable advice is highlighted in sidebars in each chapter. Recipe suggestions throughout the book will show you how to turn that advice into meals, snacks, and even treats that harness the power of your blender to uplevel your nutrition.

In Chapter 6, you will find our 7-Day Beast Blending Lifestyle Plan, which pulls together all the Fuel Up Habits we cover into a week's worth of healthy eating and hydration so you can experience what it's like to truly be fully fueled. That's followed by more than 100 additional recipes for a lot more than just smoothies, but also soups, dressings, condiments, drinks, and more to provide you with a wide variety of options for making healthy eating as easy and delicious as possible.

One last note before we get started: we hope that you will use this book to find the optimal level of healthy eating *for you.* The advice and recipes in this book are flexible enough to work with your personal goals and health status, but they are not meant to be a cure-all. If you have health challenges that could be affected by dietary changes, please consult your doctor before following our advice. And, even if you don't, make sure to monitor how your body responds and make adjustments as needed (a topic we will talk more about in the book!).

With that said, let's get cheating! And let's feel good about it while we do. ☺

Our promise to you:

- This is *not* a diet book.

- Our advice is not built on restriction or on forbidden or "bad" foods.

- There will be no blaming or shaming around your food choices.

- There is no such thing as a perfect way to eat.

- We aim, always, to make our recipes and advice as accessible and actionable as possible—for real people with real lives and real budgets to consider.

- When you eat, we want it to be an *enjoyable* experience—and we believe strongly that healthy eating can be just that!

CHAPTER 1:

Make Blending a Habit

Fuel Up Habit #1

Kick off your days with a blended meal from our Smoothies with Benefits Program.

Bethsaida was an ancient fishing village on the Sea of Galilee that makes multiple appearances in the New Testament. In the Gospel of Mark, a blind man is brought to Jesus, who leads the man out of Bethsaida before restoring his sight.[1] In the Gospel of Luke, Jesus performs a miracle by turning five loaves and two fish into enough food to feed 5,000 men who have congregated there.[2] Over time, the exact location of this biblical town has been lost to history, a fact that has inspired several present-day archaeologists to go on the hunt for it.

And some believe they have found it. The site of el-Araj, on the northeast shore of the Sea of Galilee, has been under excavation by archaeologists who believe it is Bethsaida. In 2023, Thomas G. Guilliams, Ph.D., of the Point Institute—a brilliant friend of Dr. Dana's and a leader of archaeological tours—excavated a mortar and three different pestles near a clay oven that was likely part of a small home there. The home dates to the 2nd or 3rd century CE, so the mortar and pestles would be about the same age. They are thought to have been used to grind up all sorts of foods, including grains, root vegetables, and even meat.

To us this is evidence that when we use a blender to cheat our way to optimal health, we are taking part in a longstanding tradition. Humans have been utilizing tools to crush and grind their foods for a very long time. Whereas today we have more efficient tools like a blender at our disposal, the mortar and pestle has been in use since the Stone Age to release flavor and make foods easier to combine, cook, and digest.[3]

In fact, there are so many different cooking aids to choose from these days, from air fryers to sous vide machines, that we think the humble blender often gets overlooked. And that's a shame, because its speed, efficiency, and ease of use make it a perfect tool to help almost anyone establish healthier eating habits that can last.

This doesn't mean that we're going to ask you to blend all your food, of course. Drinking all your meals would be a dull way to eat and difficult to sustain. Besides, chewing is an important part of the digestive process. In fact, many of our blender recipes—including our sauces, dressings, and condiments—are meant to be added to foods that you chew, like proteins or veggies, to optimize both their flavor and uplevel their nutritional value. We will be talking more about those kinds of recipes later in this book, but in this chapter, we're going to start off simply by asking you to use your blender to do just one thing: make your daily breakfast.

This means that, instead of whatever you typically have in the mornings, you will begin your day with a blend from what we call our Smoothies with Benefits Program. We understand that this may be a new way of eating for you and that change can be hard, especially when it comes to something as ingrained as our eating habits. That's why, after introducing you to the specially designed blends you will be choosing from for breakfast, we're going to spend the second half of this chapter helping you set yourself up so that this new habit works within the realities of *your* everyday life. We want to make this habit as easy and as pleasurable as possible. That way, it's more likely to last and make a real difference in the way that you feel.

Our Smoothies with Benefits Program

Smoothies are tasty, quick, and easy to make, which is why the Internet and social media are filled with them. But ours are not just any old smoothie recipes. They are designed to serve the specific purpose of helping you start off your day feeling vital, strong, and fully fueled.

By design, they do two very important things that not all smoothie recipes do:

1. They serve as a full meal.

A common problem with many of the smoothies you find online or purchase at your local juice bar is that they leave you feeling hungry within an hour or two. That's because they're conceived more with flavor in mind than optimal nutrition, whereas ours satisfy both!

Too often people will build a smoothie around certain ingredients that may well be healthy but then neglect to consider the total nutritional picture. We don't do that. All our Smoothies with Benefits contain a full serving of protein (about 20 grams), a healthy fat, and a generous dose of fiber, because skimping on any one of these things can leave you feeling depleted and hungry. What's more, because most of us aren't getting enough fruits and vegetables, every recipe contains at least a serving of produce, and many have much more than that. We pack all that in without overdoing the calories or, just as importantly, sacrificing flavor. Because if it doesn't taste good, what's the point? Enjoying your blended meal is a vital part of establishing this as a healthy eating habit.

2. They encourage a taste evolution.

Our Smoothies with Benefits are not just a collection of one-off recipes. They are recipes arranged on a graduating spectrum. In other words, they are designed to evolve. The first ones you encounter (in our recipe chapter, starting on page 171) will be sweeter and more fruit-forward than the rest. They highlight favorite flavors like strawberries, cocoa, banana, and pineapple. We sneak in some veggies too—like a handful of spinach or a cup of legumes—but you won't know it by the taste. They are the kind of smoothies even kids with picky palates will love.

Gradually, the flavor profile of our smoothies becomes more complex and more vegetable-forward. At the far end of the spectrum, you will even find a few not-for-the-faint-of-heart options, including one of Colin's favorites, Green Slime, which includes fresh produce from his garden like kale, Swiss chard, beets (beet greens included), and even tomatoes. Sometimes he even likes to add a shot of spirulina, a blue-green algae that, while highly nutritious, lends a dark green color and a bitter flavor that makes it something of an acquired taste.

That's what Colin likes best these days, but remember, he was the guy who started out hating the taste of vegetables. Now, he has a veggie-packed smoothie every day. And that's exactly why we have arranged our recipes in this way. Just because you don't like certain healthy foods—or maybe even *any* healthy foods—doesn't mean it has to be that way forever.

All the recipes in this book are healthy. Some may pack in more nutritional benefits than others, however, and our intention is for you to eat as healthfully as possible within the context of what works for you, which is why our Smoothie with Benefits Program offers you different smoothie levels to try. You may never learn to like spirulina, even in a blend with other ingredients to mitigate the taste, and that's fine. But then again, maybe you will! And either way, through the process of trying our different levels, you will be adding vital nutrients and finding healthy choices that you enjoy, ones that you can return to again and again.

Training Your Taste Buds

Did you know that when most people try tomatoes for the first time, they don't like the taste?[4] As a basic ingredient in American staples like red sauce and pizza, it's hard to imagine that, once upon a time, we probably didn't like this popular ingredient ourselves, but it's true. This is an example of how our tastes can change, which, when it comes to the goal of eating healthier, is a fact that can be empowering.

As you make your way through this book, you will find all sorts of ways to make healthy eating work for you—for your lifestyle, for your values, and for your tastes. One of those ways is by finding out if the healthy foods you avoid are really so unpalatable after all. Or, if you had them prepared in a certain way, is it possible that you could actually enjoy them? It's important to remember that our tastes can evolve, and there's even evidence that we can do things to help them evolve in a healthier direction.

What we're talking about here is sort of like training your taste buds. The tactics that can help you do this will work better for some people than others. We just ask that you give them a try and see what happens. After all, what do you have to lose?

One such tactic is **repeated exposure**, meaning you can sometimes develop a taste for something by trying small portions over time. This can work because familiarity is one of the key factors in determining taste—so much so that studies suggest that even the mere act of showing children pictures of different fruits and vegetables has the potential to increase their willingness to eat them.[5]

Our taste buds are often suspicious of new flavors for good reason. Back when our ancestors had to hunt and forage for food, they had to figure out for themselves, through a rather precarious process of trial and error, which plants were worth eating and which ones were poisonous. That means an unfamiliar taste could be a sign of something potentially sinister. Many people have a natural aversion to bitter-tasting foods, for example, because bitterness can be a sign of toxicity or spoiled food. Remarkably, there are bitter receptors all over our bodies, not just on our tongues, and it is believed that genetic variables among those receptors are the reason why some of us, like Colin, are supertasters who are more sensitive to the flavor.[6]

Bitters are fascinating molecules, really, produced by plants to protect them from herbivores. While they can be toxic in some cases, in others, the same qualities that protect plants can benefit us as well. Evidence suggests that bitter substances may help regulate metabolic function and specifically aid in satiation and blood sugar regulation.[7] Thankfully, unlike our ancestors, we no longer have to guess which plants fall into which category. In fact, the bitter foods we find at the supermarket—like citrus peel, cocoa, coffee, and cruciferous vegetables like broccoli and kale—typically have lots of health benefits. Unfortunately, we no longer eat as many bitter things as we used to, and the bitter foods we do eat are often not as potent as they once were. Humans have bred out the bitter flavor in many foods like arugula and endive, thereby reducing their healthfulness. That said, these foods still have plenty of benefits and are certainly worth trying more than once to see if you can develop a taste for them!

Another tactic we can try to train our taste buds is to **create positive associations** by pairing healthy foods with ones you already like—something that is easily done through blending. (See The Bitter Experiment in the following sidebar.) Dr. Dana once heard Dr. Terry Wahls, author and clinical professor of medicine at the University of Iowa, describe how she helps skeptics realize that it is possible to enjoy bitter foods. She uses dandelion greens, which have a very sharp flavor, and starts by having the person place a few ribbons on their tongues. As the bitter flavor sinks in, the typical first reaction is "Yuck!"

Next, Wahls blends the greens with grapes, a little olive oil, and ice. The fat in the olive oil helps mellow the bitterness, and the grapes add sweetness. When offering people a taste of dandelion prepared in this way, most agree that it's a totally different experience, and many even find that they like it. There is some evidence to suggest that our tastes can change to favor healthier foods using tactics like these.[8] In other words, the more we eat healthy foods, the more likely we are to enjoy eating healthy foods.

You can use your morning Smoothie with Benefits to try both these tactics. When you see an ingredient in one of our recipes that you're less fond of, consider trying it anyway, especially if it's paired with flavors you know you enjoy. For many people, this will be some sort of vegetable like spinach or kale. We had one recipe tester who had always hated lentils—until he had them in our **Lovely Lentil Brownie Bites** (page 211). Not only did the lentils make the treat nutrient dense and full of protein, when prepared in this way, he was surprised to find that they tasted great too!

The Bitter Experiment

Try a version of Dr. Terry Wahls's bitter-flavor experiment for yourself.

1. Choose a bitter vegetable. Dandelion greens, collards, endive, or radicchio are all good options.

2. Try placing a bit of the raw vegetable on your tongue, maybe even chewing it a little, so you understand the flavor profile you're working with.

3. Next, blend the vegetable with a splash of olive oil and something sweet. Wahls used grapes with her dandelion greens, but you can also try collards with banana and berries, endive with apple, radicchio with mango, or whatever combination inspires you. (Note: you may need to add a little water if the ingredients don't blend easily.)

4. You can also try cooking the vegetables in a little bit of olive oil to mellow the flavor. Other options for dressing up bitter flavors include adding an acid, like lemon juice or vinegar, and/or adding spices with heat, like red pepper flakes or chili powder.

5. Note how different combinations and preparation methods affect flavor and consider using that knowledge going forward to try new foods, or to retry old ones that you have previously written off.

To Build Habits That Last, Know Your Why

There are a lot of fad diets and trendy health advice out there, and most of the recommendations do not produce lasting change, which is why we are focused on helping to make the basic principles of healthy eating easier and more sustainable—using your blender as your ultimate cheating tool. Remember what we said in the opening of this book: healthy eating shouldn't be so hard.

This doesn't mean that changing some things about how you eat isn't going to be challenging at times. So, when building a new habit, what helps? What can you do to make it as easy as possible to sustain?

One thing that can be useful is to spend some time thinking about your *why*. You bought this book and are reading it now for a reason. What is it? The obvious answer might be "to get healthier," but let's take that thought a little further. What is your motivation for wanting to get or stay healthy?

One of Dr. Dana's all-time favorite books is *Man's Search for Meaning* by the Holocaust survivor and psychiatrist Viktor Frankl. In it, he wrote about how he believed there were commonalities among those who survived the concentration camps. The way he saw it, they were typically people who had a strong sense of purpose and who could imagine how that purpose connected to the future they envisioned for themselves beyond their current circumstances.

Our lives are very different from Frankl's, of course, but our motivations still matter. So, what are yours? Ask yourself: *What would feeling healthier allow me to do in my life? How might my life be different as a result?*

When we asked these kinds of questions of people who tried a version of our Beast Blending Lifestyle Plan, which you'll learn about in Chapter 6, we got some expected answers and some less expected ones too. "For my kids" or "for my family" were among the most common, with some repeating the familiar sentiment that they wanted to be around long enough to dance at their grandchildren's weddings. Career was another big one. Colin says he always makes a point of starting his day off with a nutrient-packed smoothie because he's come to realize that he needs it to have the kind of energy and self-belief required to run his own business. Others talked about their hobbies, their passion for things like travel or public service, even their pets. For Dr. Dana, staying healthy allows her to help more people, and she believes there is nothing more fulfilling than when someone tells her they feel so much better because of her advice.

A number of people also talked about their current health status and how it sometimes got in the way of living their lives to the fullest. Maybe they'd had a health scare like a heart attack or cancer, or maybe they had been diagnosed with a chronic illness like diabetes or an auto-immune condition. Still others were just tired of feeling depleted and not at their best most of the time. Whether out of fear or frustration or both, these people were looking for a way to feel better, healthier, and more vital so they could enjoy their lives more and stress about their health less.

There are no wrong answers here. Maybe some of these examples strike a chord in you, or maybe you have reasons that are entirely your own. The key thing here is that the answer resonates with you. Your personal reason for wanting to get healthier is something you can revisit as you make your way through this book, building more and more healthy eating habits along the way.

And if you can't think of a *why* that feels big enough, just start any-way. Follow our advice for building healthy habits and see what happens. We find that doing so creates a kind of snowball effect. Once people try starting their day with a nutrient-packed smoothie, they typically begin to feel the difference it can make quite quickly—in their energy lev-els, their mood, their confidence, and their overall sense of health and well-being—and that feeling is its own kind of motivation. When people start feeling better, they want to continue to feel better, and sticking to the habit, and then building on it, becomes easier as a result.

Case Study: Dr. Christine

Dr. Christine came at this from a unique perspective. "As a mom and a doctor, I know it's really important to eat healthy," she explained. "I know what I *should* be eating, and that includes healthy servings of vegetables and fruits every day. But that doesn't always happen."

Dr. Christine had some real hurdles that she knew she had to overcome. First, being both a mom and a doctor meant that she had a very busy lifestyle, one that wasn't conducive to spending a lot of time in the kitchen preparing healthy food. The other was perhaps even trickier. She hated vegetables—so much so, she says, "I would even pick the peas out of my fried rice."

As part of a new eating program, she started using her blender every single day to make a Smoothie with Benefits for breakfast. The program (a version of which you will find in Chapter 6) also guided her to take hydration breaks and enjoy other healthy meals and snacks throughout the day, but it was that morning blend that made the biggest difference. She said it allowed her "to get those vegetables in that I don't like to eat in a way that is quick, efficient, and tastes delicious."

After just a few weeks, she was feeling so much better—both physically and mentally—that she was ready to turn her morning Smoothie with Benefits into a regular habit and committed to continuing the practice "indefinitely."

She felt motivated to do so because, as she explained it: "I feel like I can conquer the world and conquer the day!"

Make It Easy: Tips for Setting Yourself Up for Success

When establishing a new habit, no matter what it is, there is one very important factor that experts counsel people to focus on: How can you make it *easier* on yourself to *stick* to the habit?[9]

This is known as "reducing friction," which basically means reducing the amount of time and effort it takes to engage in a desired behavior. Some common examples are to choose a gym that's a short distance from your house or lay out your gym clothes before you go to bed at night (or maybe even sleep in them!) if getting in a workout first thing in the morning is your goal. When it comes to eating healthy, using your blender to cheat your way to good health is all about reducing friction. It's fast. It's easy. You don't need to practice or take a cooking class to master it. It's a low-friction solution.

When it comes to making blending a daily habit, we can take the idea of reducing friction even further by anticipating some of the obstacles you might come up against. Then we will engage in some counterprogramming to minimize or even remove those obstacles entirely before they have a chance to get in your way. In other words, we plan ahead to make the habit of starting your day with a Smoothie with Benefits as easy as possible.

What follows are some of the most common problems reported by people who have tried our Smoothies with Benefits Program and how we have helped them navigate—or *cheat* their way around—those obstacles. Use them to think through what might get in your way and how you can set yourself up for success.

The Problem: "I don't have time to eat healthy."

The Cheat: Breakfast in five minutes.

This is by far the most common thing we hear from people, but we promise you do have time for this. A healthy and delicious Smoothie with Benefits breakfast can be made in just five minutes, which is not much longer than it takes to make a piece of toast. (Yes, we timed it.) And you can do it in even less time if you set yourself up using the following strategies:

Set up your blending station.

A little preparation goes a long way, as the saying goes. When starting a meditation practice, for example, one of the first things you're told to do is to set up your practice space. This means choosing a place that will work for this purpose—i.e., away from distractions—and place there everything you will need for your practice, whether that's pillows or a mat, speakers if you like background music, and maybe even a candle or some incense. This way, when it comes time to meditate, all you have to do is sit down in your space and get started.

To create a blending habit, we suggest you do the same: Set up a space in your kitchen so that your morning routine is as accessible as possible. Clear an area on your countertop where your blender can live—permanently. That way you don't have to pull it out every morning to use it. If you use a cutting board, knife, and measuring utensils, set them out too—if you even need them. You can also bypass the need for additional equipment by using pre-prepped ingredients (see the next strategy) and simply eyeballing a couple handfuls of berries, a glassful of liquid, and so on. Blending is very forgiving this way.

Prep ahead of time.

As you unload your groceries, take a little extra time to prep any produce you will use in your smoothies for the week. This means pre-washing, pre-peeling, and precutting any ingredients that require it. This way, when morning comes, all you have to do is toss the ingredients in your blender. No work. No hassle. Just quick and easy.

If even that sounds like too much trouble, buy prewashed and pre-chopped produce. Or buy frozen, which is already cleaned, prepped, and cut into blender-size pieces. Plus, it is often cheaper than fresh fruits and veggies. It's the cheatiest of cheats!

Best Way to Clean Your Produce

All produce should be washed before eating, and the following instructions for a quick baking soda bath work best to remove pesticide residue.[10] (Note: Soap, bleach, or commercial produce washes are not recommended, because they can leave residues of their own, which you may ingest.)

1. Use 1 teaspoon of baking soda per 2 cups of cold water. Swirl the water around until the baking soda has dissolved.

2. Submerge produce in the baking soda bath, moving it around a bit to ensure that all sides get clean. Let it soak for at least 8 minutes, and up to 15 for even better cleaning.

3. For firm produce like apples, potatoes, or carrots, you can also use a soft bristle brush to give them a scrub.

4. Remove the produce from the bath and make sure it's dry before storing.

Bundle your ingredients.

After cleaning and prepping, store your smoothie ingredients all together in one place. We like to use a plastic storage bin with a tight-fitting lid for ingredients that go in the fridge, like fresh fruit, greens, ginger, or herbs. This way, all we have to do is pull out the bin in the morning, and we have everything we need without having to hunt for it. It's also a great way to keep produce fresh longer, since most refrigerated produce stays fresher when sealed. We use a similar bin for frozen smoothie ingredients and a basket for items that are stored in the pantry, like seeds, nut butters, cocoa powder, Colin's spirulina, maybe some canned pumpkin. It takes the thinking out of our morning smoothie prep.

This is also a great way to cut down on food waste. Your smoothie bin can become a place where you put items that you want to use up. Have leftover parsley or basil from last night's dinner? Unused veggies or uneaten fruits that are a little past their prime? Things that you would typically throw away, like beet greens and carrot tops? Toss them in the bin to add to your blends. Even leftover oatmeal, cooked lentils, and other cooked grains like quinoa and millet work well in smoothies. As you get into the habit of making blends on a regular basis, it will become easier to eyeball ingredients and decide what works to provide the flavor and consistency you're looking for. And this is true for more than just smoothies, but also sauces, soups, dressings, and more. You can use this practice to uplevel the nutrients *and* cut down on waste at the same time.

Try our **The Perfect Pumpkin Breakfast Bowl** (page 181) to use up cooked grains like oatmeal or our **"Trash Can" Poaching Broth** (page 193) to use up common throwaway items like carrot tops, broccoli stems, and beet greens.

Make it to go.

Digestion works best when we're relaxed, so ideally, we would all sit down to eat our breakfast without distractions and take time to savor our food. The Buddhist Zen master Thich Nhat Hanh, who wrote a charmingly illustrated book about mindful eating, put it this way: "When we can slow down and really enjoy our food, our life takes on a much deeper quality." He even had a verse he liked to recite when he ate, which starts like this:

In the dimension of space and time,
We chew as rhythmically as we breathe.[11]

This is a lovely ideal and one we hope you will aim for when you can. However, we live in the real world too and often find ourselves eating on the go, which can be stressful. It helps a lot if our on-the-go meal is a healthy one, which is not always easy since most fast food is anything but. Smoothies, however, are a highly portable fast-food option—much more so than a bowl of oatmeal or a plate of eggs—and they're good for you too. So, if you know you will be pressed for time in the morning, set yourself up to have your smoothie to go. Beast makes a drinking lid and carry cap with a handle for this purpose, but if you don't have one, buy yourself a commuter cup so you can enjoy your smoothie while you're in the car, on the subway, at the office, or walking your kids to school. It's not quite what Thich Nhat Hanh would recommend, but it's good enough to get you through a busy morning. And we bet that even he ate on the road once in a while!

The Problem: "I didn't get to the grocery store this week."

The Cheat: Stock up so you're always smoothie ready.

Life gets overwhelming sometimes, and every one of us has weeks when we don't get to the grocery store because we run out of time, or we don't feel up to it for one reason or another. We love the taste of fresh produce in our smoothies, but you can still make healthy and delicious breakfast blends entirely out of nonperishable items from your freezer and pantry. With just a little forethought, you can ensure that you always have on hand what you need to make a healthy breakfast.

Following is a list of items that we recommend you keep in stock for your smoothies. These are just some basics, so feel free to add any favorites to the list.

Smoothie-Ready Items

- Frozen berries of your choice (or any other favorite fruit)
- Peeled and sliced frozen bananas (to add creamy texture)
- Frozen greens like spinach or kale (for added nutrients)

- Nonperishable proteins like seeds, nuts, nut butters, frozen peas, or frozen edamame (to provide energy and keep you feeling full)
- Nonperishable milk substitute like almond or soy (water works too)
- Maybe one of Dr. Dana's protein powders or your own favorite brand (see Resources)

Your freezer can be one of your best assets when you want to make sure that you always have healthy options on hand. It's also a great way to cut down on food waste. Have some bananas that are browning fast? Peel and cut into blender-ready slices before freezing. Berries in danger of turning fuzzy? Freeze them. There are even some blender-ready items that unexpectedly freeze well, like slices of avocado or knuckles of ginger, which can be grated from frozen straight into your blender.

You can even cheat on this cheat! Check the frozen-food section of your grocery store for prepackaged smoothie ingredients, which are already cleaned, chopped, portioned, and ready to blend. Dr. Dana's favorite is Costco Smoothie Packs by Clovis Farms, which offer six packages of smoothie-ready fruits and vegetables for about $12. She prefers to make her own blends most days, but these are great in a pinch. She often adds a handful of spinach or kale, or leftover herbs like parsley if she has it, just to boost the nutrient content.

> Try our **Edamam-Yay!** (page 177) or **Quick and Tasty** (page 175) recipes to make Smoothies with Benefits entirely out of nonperishable items from your freezer or pantry.

The Problem: "I don't have all the ingredients I need for the recipe I want to make."

The Cheat: Make substitutions freely.

One of the best things about blending as a healthy eating strategy is that it's highly versatile. Recipes don't have to be followed to the letter, and ingredients don't have to be measured precisely. If a recipe calls for something you don't have or can't find at the store, then swap it for something comparable. You can do the same with ingredients that you really don't care for, though we hope you will give your taste buds a chance to learn to love them before you do.

Some easy swaps include:

- If our recipe calls for blueberries . . .
- Swap them for any other berry, a mix of berries, or even a comparable amount of another fruit like grapes, mango chunks, or stone fruit.
- If our recipe calls for almond milk . . .
- Swap it for any other type of milk that works for you, from cow's milk to soy, macadamia, oat, rice, seed (like flax or hemp), or any of the many milk substitutes that are on the market these days. Water also works.
- If our recipe calls for Greek yogurt . . .
- Swap it for something that offers a comparable amount of protein and also adds thickness, like nondairy yogurt or silken tofu (good options if you're lactose intolerant), or even cottage cheese or ricotta.
- If our recipe calls for spinach . . .
- Swap it for just about any leafy green like kale, Swiss chard, romaine, arugula, watercress, or even some more unusual items like mizuna or komatsuna.
- If our recipe calls for hemp seeds . . .
- Swap it for a comparable amount of flax, chia, or sesame seeds, or a seed blend. The same advice holds true for any nut or nut butter that we recommend.

The Problem: "I don't want to clean my blender every day."

The Cheat: Quick-clean strategies.

Because we're asking you to use your blender daily, you're going to want to know how to keep it clean without a lot of hassle. After all, if it's sitting in the sink waiting to be washed, you will be that much less motivated to start your morning with a healthy blend.

Many blending vessels like the Beast are designed to be dishwasher safe (check the manufacturer's details to be sure), but that doesn't do you much good unless you run your dishwasher every day. Instead, we recommend that you run it through the dishwasher once a week and then use one of our quick-clean strategies daily. You have two options:

1. Fill the vessel with warm water and a drop or two of dish soap. Pulse it a few times until the water gets soapy, then empty it and rinse. Leave it to dry next to your blending station so it's ready for tomorrow.

2. Colin's preferred method is even faster: he uses warm water and a cleaning brush to give it a quick scrub before leaving it to dry for the next morning.

Doing this *immediately after use* is key to avoiding stuck-on foods. While you clean your blender, remember to rinse off your knife, cutting board, and measuring utensils, if you used them, and leave them out to dry. The idea is to ensure you have as little to do in the morning when you might be bleary-eyed and short on time.

The Problem: "I don't want a cold smoothie every day. Sometimes I want something hot to eat!"

The Cheat: Warm smoothie bowls

Sometimes a cold smoothie on a cold day just isn't what you are craving. And that's completely understandable. Dr. Dana often has the same reaction on wintry days! Which is why we have provided you with some warm breakfast options in the form of porridges—warm, cooked grains like quinoa, millet, or oatmeal—with pour-over smoothies for added nutrients and flavor. You will find those options starting on page 181.

The Problem: "Sometimes I want to go out to brunch with my friends!"

The Cheat: Pregaming Smoothies

Please do go out with your friends! We will simply suggest some ways to fuel yourself before you do, a practice we like to call *pregaming*. The term typically refers to the habit of getting tipsy before going out on the town, but we give it a healthy twist, of course. We use it to refer to a practice we recommend of gifting yourself and your body with a dose of nutrients and hydration *before* you head out to brunch, or anywhere else—like a cocktail party, business lunch, or holiday meal—where you know the fare won't be the healthiest. You can do this by downing one of what we call our Salad Shooters, which are three-gulp smoothies packed with goodness to help prepare you for what's to come.

We will talk more about this practice in Chapter 3, when we discuss how to maximize the variety of plant foods you enjoy throughout the day, but for now just know that we would never ask you to stay home for the sake of your breakfast. Socializing is important. In fact, recent research on the link between loneliness and serious health conditions shows that it's even more important than many of us realized.[12] We would never ask you to give up your favorite foods unless there was a really important reason to, like a food allergy. What is the point of learning to fuel yourself better if it leads to enjoying your life less? Our aim is to help you do both!

The Problem: "I can't make a smoothie when I'm traveling."

The Cheat: Travel Smoothies

Colin actually travels with his blender. No joke. Many personal blenders are quite compact on their own, and the Beast even comes in a travel size. Colin packs his in a portable cooler bag alongside ziplock bags filled with seeds for protein and heartier produce like carrots, celery, cucumber, broccoli, and/or kale leaves. He uses juice or even just water from the hotel as his liquid, and voilà! He has enough to make smoothies in his room for several days.

This is a great option for people who travel a lot like Colin does, but if it's not something you can see yourself doing, then plan ahead. Look up nearby juice bars, local smoothie shops, restaurants, or even health-food and grocery stores. The thing you want to remember is to check the ingredients before you buy. Many smoothies are packed with things you don't need, like added sugars, and don't have enough of what you do need, like protein. Use our Smoothies with Benefits as a guide and try to find something similar.

Enjoy Your Food: It's Good for Your Health

As a final word on the subject of making blending a habit, we want to emphasize that one of the best and most sustainable healthy eating strategies is to like what you eat. And we're not just telling you that because it's what you want to hear. It may sound like something of a contradiction, but eating for pleasure has been linked to making *better* nutritional choices, not worse ones.[13, 14]

It's for this reason that one of our primary goals throughout this book is to make healthy food taste good. Of course, taste is highly personal, which is why we offer a range of options with different flavor profiles in each of our recipe categories—so you have choices. As you build your smoothie-a-day habit, we suggest you start with something you know you will like. Focus on what's going to make it easiest and most enjoyable for you to get up and *want* to have that smoothie each day. We offer a couple of popular options at the end of this chapter, but feel free to choose anything from the Smoothies with Benefits section of Chapter 7.

And remember that enjoying your food can be about more than just flavor. "You eat with your eyes first," as the old saying goes, so think about presentation. If it appeals to you, dress up your smoothie by putting a cherry on top or a dusting of cinnamon, or by serving it in a special glass. You can use frozen ingredients and add a little less liquid to make the texture thick and milkshake-y so it feels decadent to drink. In our recipe chapter, you will find directions on how to turn any of our smoothies into smoothie bowls if you find it more fun to eat them that way. (See the sidebar for a list of healthy flavor additives you can use to top any smoothie or smoothie bowl.)

And don't forget about color! Social media is filled with brightly hued smoothie images for a reason, so make your morning blend Instagrammable if you like. Lots of healthy ingredients make for pretty pictures. Cooked beets can make for a beautiful, dark-red smoothie (and add a bit of sweetness at the same time). Dragon fruit is good for frothy pink versions. Turmeric turns things bright orange. (And, as you will read about in Chapter 3, colorful plants have health benefits too!)

Healthy Flavor Additives

- A sprinkling of natural cocoa powder or cacao nibs

- Chopped nuts like pecans, almonds, walnuts, or pistachios

- A dusting of cinnamon

- Shredded or flaked coconut

- A handful of berries

- Pomegranate seeds

- Diced apple

- Dried fruits like raisins or currants

- Fresh mint leaves

Another way to level up your enjoyment is to get others involved. Make your morning smoothie preparation into a ritual that you do with your partner or kids. Or taste-test different recipes with a friend, giving you an excuse to check in with each other on a daily basis. Go ahead and post those Instagrammable smoothies to get your community involved if you want to (and don't forget to tag us!). Or do none of these things if you're not a morning person and just want to drink your smoothie in peace. The point is to think about what's going to make this habit work best for you, not just tomorrow but for mornings to come.

In this chapter, we've asked you to do just one thing: have your first meal be a Smoothie with Benefits. We have given you lots of ideas and advice for making that work, but ultimately how it fits into your life is up to you! And in the next chapter, we'll talk about how to make health*ier* choices when you get to the grocery store so you can start thinking about how best to fuel yourself through the rest of your day.

Recipes to Try Today!
Smoothies with Benefits That
Practically Everyone Will Love

Directions for making your Smoothie with Benefits. Both options are from our Level 1: Starter Smoothies category and make 1 serving.

1. Add all ingredients to your blender.

2. Blend until smooth, about 1 minute.

3. Enjoy!

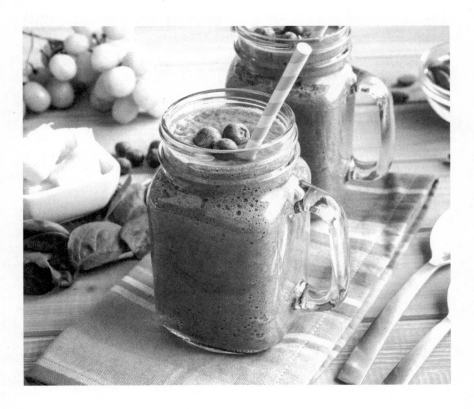

THE SUPREME PROTEIN SMOOTHIE

If you're a fan of tropical fruit flavors, this is a great option to start with. It's also a good choice if you're an active person or if you tend to get hungry again soon after eating, because it's packed with protein. Soy milk, edamame, hemp seeds, and Greek yogurt all serve this purpose, with the yogurt also adding a tangy zip!

1 cup unsweetened soy milk
1 cup frozen shelled edamame
½ cup Greek yogurt
¼ cup pineapple chunks
¼ banana
1 teaspoon hemp seeds
Handful of ice (optional)

SIMPLY DELICIOUS

If you like the ease and flavor of protein powder, this is a good place to start. (We use Dr. Dana's brand, of course, but you can choose your favorite.) The flavor of berries mixed with your choice of chocolate or vanilla is sure to please practically any palate.

1 cup unsweetened nut, seed, or oat milk
½ banana
¼ cup blueberries
¼ cup strawberries
1 cup spinach
1 serving protein powder
Handful of ice (optional)

Cheat Sheet

3 Ways to Get into a Blending Habit . . . Right Away!

1. **Try Your First Smoothie with Benefits Today!**
   Choose something that sounds delicious. We have suggested a couple of options, but you can pick any recipe in the Smoothie with Benefits section starting on page 173. Then make a plan for the rest of the week. Will you have the same smoothie every day, or do you want to try different options? Do what works for you!

2. **Define Your Why**
   Take some time to think about *why* you want to start eating in a healthier way. Imagine what life will be like and what it will enable you to do. You might even write down your *why* and post it or keep it somewhere that you can revisit as you make your way through the rest of this book.

3. **Set Yourself Up for Success**
   Try to anticipate some of the obstacles that might get in the way of your new smoothie-a-day habit, and then engage in some counterprogramming: What can you do today that will make keeping this habit easier and more enjoyable in the coming days?

CHAPTER 2

Consume More Foods as Nature Intended

Fuel Up Habit #2

Start shifting the balance in your eating patterns
to favor more natural (and often yummier!)
options and fewer ultraprocessed foods (UPFs).

As we have said before: Nutrition advice can be so complicated! Especially when you get to the grocery store and have to translate all the different messages you have heard from your doctor, from the media, and from friends and family into what to actually buy so you can feed yourself.

You may be aware, for example, that most Americans don't get enough fiber. Maybe you have even had some GI issues, and your doctor said that more fiber could help. She told you to aim for 25 grams a day. Great! But what does that mean when dinnertime comes around and you need to put something on the table before you and the rest of the family start to get hangry? What does 25 grams of fiber even look like?

One of the best strategies we can offer you is to forget about counting calories or trying to calculate nutritional information from the back of packaging. Unless you love to do that sort of thing (and who does, really?), it can make the act of eating well feel like a chore—difficult, confusing, and time-consuming—which is a great way to sabotage any healthy intention. That's why the advice we're going to cover in this chapter is the opposite of that. In fact, it could not be more straightforward: simply focus on eating more foods as nature intended.

So, what does that mean? We will go into it in depth in this chapter, but generally speaking it means upleveling your nutrition by choosing real, whole foods over processed or packaged options whenever and wherever possible. That doesn't mean you have to do it all the time or feel bad when you do choose packaged foods. In fact, *some* packaged and processed foods are even good for you. In this chapter, we will help clarify the differences by breaking things down, minimizing the noise, and showing you how your blender can help you simplify the task of eating more real food.

Why Food "As Nature Intended"?

This advice works because Mother Nature has our backs. Everything our bodies need to thrive, from the macronutrients (protein, carbs, fats) to the micronutrients (all the different vitamins and minerals), can be found in nature. She has a pretty pleasing way of offering them to us too. Have you ever been to a farmer's market and marveled at the sheer variety—colors, shapes, sizes, and textures—of ingredients that can nourish us?

Of course, farms are not the only place where we get our food these days. Much, if not most, of what we eat comes not from a farm but from a factory or a processing plant. We promised in the opening to this book not to act as the food police or to demonize particular foods, but there is one general category to watch out for, and we would be remiss if we didn't mention it: ultraprocessed foods (UPFs).

In our view, UPFs are the opposite of real, as-nature-intended foods. They can be defined as "industrially manufactured, ready-to-eat or ready-to-heat formulations . . . with little, if any, whole foods."[1] They often contain additives like colorings, flavorings, sweeteners, preservatives, and emulsifiers.[2] Think sodas and energy drinks, packaged snack chips and puffs, and many kinds of frozen, microwavable meals, to name just a few examples. What's more, industrial processing can change the structure of food to the point where it becomes what some describe as essentially "predigested" (ick!).[3] In other words, UPFs are items that contain "little if any intact food."[4] It's like Jerry Seinfeld's old joke about the Pop-Tart: "They can't go stale, because they were never fresh in the first place."[5] It's the kind of thing you would never find in nature.

Why does this matter? Because a wide body of research shows that a diet high in UPFs is correlated with an increased risk of serious health conditions, including metabolic syndrome, cardiovascular disease, cancer, type 2 diabetes, irritable bowel syndrome, and frailty.[6, 7] Most people haven't heard much about that last one, but frailty is a condition common among older people that has become a strong predictor of negative outcomes, like longer hospital stays, nursing home placement, and even death.[8] On top of all of that, high rates of UPF consumption have been generally associated with a greater risk of death from any cause, and that's not something we should ignore.

Our brains may also be affected. More recent research has focused on this area, including a 2022 cohort study that found a connection between UPFs and a higher rate of cognitive decline among middle-aged and older adults.[9] These findings held true across genders and diverse ethnic backgrounds. There have also been studies linking high UPF consumption to depression.[10]

Exactly how a diet high in UPFs might lead to something like heart disease, for example, is an area that's still being studied. What we do know, however, is that foods in this category tend to be much higher in things we want to eat in moderation, like less healthy fats, sodium, and sugar. Processing foods can also strip out important nutrients, leaving behind a product with a lower concentration of things our bodies need, like vitamins, minerals, and fiber. What's more, UPFs are generally hyperpalatable (i.e., super tasty!) by design, which means they can promote cravings and overeating to the point where some even call them addictive. [11, 12] Certain food additives, present only in processed foods, potentially play a role by altering the bacteria in our microbiomes, increasing inflammation and other potential consequences.[13, 14]

And these are just some of the ways UPFs can impact your health. It's a topic that could fill the pages of an entire book if we really got into the science, but what's really important for most of us to know is that, when deciding what to buy at the grocery store, it's worth paying attention to just how much of your food is ultraprocessed.

With all that said, we want you to understand that we are not telling you to *never* eat UPFs. There is too much demonizing of food in our culture, especially in the press and on social media, and that's not our aim here. If a person who is relatively healthy reaches for a bag of chips once in a while, or a store-bought coffee cake with 40-plus ingredients, it's not going to kill them. Nor is it healthy to make people feel guilty about these kinds of choices. Instead, what we want to focus on here is how you can **make healthier choices more often**.

As it turns out, there's a lot of opportunity to make healthier choices when it comes to UPFs. In the U.S., UPFs account for a surprisingly high percentage of our total calories: as much as 57 percent,[15] with some estimates putting it even higher.[16, 17] And that number remains consistently high across various demographics, including different education and income levels,[18] which means that just about all of us can find room to uplevel some, if not many, of our food choices.

Imagine a scale with foods as nature intended on one side and UPFs on the other. If you are like most people, then that scale is currently tipped in favor of UPFs. What we are going to do in this chapter is start tipping the scale in the other direction. You don't need to worry about being perfect, just about shifting the balance in nature's favor. Starting from wherever you are—regardless of whether you eat lots of UPFs or just a few—we are going to look for ways you can make healthier choices without feeling like you are depriving yourself. We want to do this because UPFs tend to be lower-quality fuel for our bodies. When we swap them out for higher-quality fuel, it can not only help protect you from disease, but also help you feel better on a daily basis.

Case Study: Richard

For Richard, a security professional in his 60s, one of his top health goals was to age well: to do what he could to ensure that he lived a long and healthy life—one where he continued to feel strong, capable, and independent well into his twilight years.

- He wanted to change the way he ate because he knew that his current habits didn't entirely support that goal. "I was very busy," he explained. "The pandemic had ended, and I was out and about. I was eating a lot of junk food. There was a lot of snacking." Ice cream was a favorite. As were potato chips. And like many of us, he knew he wasn't eating enough vegetables.

- To jump-start the change, he decided to try a new eating plan for 30 days. He started every morning with a Smoothie with Benefits, which was packed with the veggies he had been missing. Then he used our recipes to eat more foods as nature intended throughout the rest of the day. Focusing on just those things made a real difference.

- "I think my taste buds have changed, because I'm not craving any crap," he said at the end of it. He had eliminated most ultraprocessed foods and fast foods from his diet because he just didn't feel like he wanted them as much and he had satisfying alternatives to put in their place. He could tell that these changes had made a real difference.

- Richard said he just felt better. He had more energy. His sleep had improved. He even said, "I'm a lot stronger than I was thirty days ago." It also felt good to know that he was doing his best to continue to be active and healthy well into the future.

What Does "As Nature Intended" Mean Exactly?

Real foods. Whole foods. As-nature-intended foods. What do these (relatively interchangeable) terms mean when you get to the grocery store and start filling up your cart?

It's important to be able to distinguish between this category, which you want more of, and UPFs, which you want less of so that you can start tipping the scale in nature's favor. Often, it can be quite easy. A carrot is real food, obviously. On the other hand, a store-bought, cream-cheese-frosted carrot cake sold in a plastic clamshell with a label listing an imposing block of ingredients is a UPF. Not a difficult distinction there.

But it's not always so simple. In between those two extremes is a whole spectrum of carroty options, from less processed to more. Peeled and shredded raw carrots. Frozen carrots. Sliced, canned carrots. Carrot juice. Packaged carrot-ginger soup. Frozen honey-glazed carrots. A microwavable meal of pot roast and roasted carrots. All are processed to some degree. So, how much processing is too much?

In fact, researchers make a distinction between *ultra*processed foods and simply processed or packaged ones. Because, let's face it, just about everything you find in the grocery store has been "processed" to some degree. Chicken, for example, is never just chicken when you're shopping. You might buy a whole chicken, or chicken pieces that the butcher has cut up for you, or meat that has already been skinned, deboned, or even ground. All of it has been processed in a way (otherwise, it would come with the feathers still on), but this isn't the kind of processing we are concerned about.

To help people distinguish among the different levels of processing, researchers at the University of São Paulo, Brazil, came up with the **NOVA Food Classification System.** Recognized by the World Health Organization, it identifies four levels that range from barely to highly processed foods:[19]

1. Unprocessed or minimally processed foods

This includes your basic, single-ingredient foods like carrots or chicken. It also includes anything that has been altered only slightly, but the original, as-nature-intended ingredient is still intact enough that the nutrition content has not substantially changed. So, that carrot can be peeled and cut into carrot sticks, or that chicken can be ground.

Examples include:

Fresh and frozen fruits and veggies

Fresh and dried mushrooms

Juices with no added ingredients, like sugar

Whole grains like oats and rice

Dried beans and legumes

Raw or roasted nuts and seeds without added salt or sugar

Fresh and dried herbs and spices

Pasteurized milk and plain yogurt

Eggs

Fresh and frozen meats, fish, or seafood

2. Processed culinary ingredients

This category includes ingredients that are used in cooking or baking rather than eaten on their own, like oils, fats, salt, flours, and other starches. They, too, are minimally processed, usually through methods like pressing, milling, grinding, or refining. When used in moderation to create your own dishes, they are generally healthy options. There are some ingredients in this category, however, that you will want to use more sparingly, like sugars and excess fats, especially trans fats.

Examples of processed culinary foods include:

Oils derived from plants, like olive and avocado oil

Real honey and maple syrup

Starches from tapioca, corn, and other plants

Flours made from wheat, almond, or other plants

Salts

The Truth about Trans Fats

Despite the bad rap that fats sometimes get, they are an essential macronutrient that our bodies require. And yet, not all fats are equal. Trans-fatty acids, commonly called trans fats, are especially worth paying attention to because they significantly increase your risk of heart disease, diabetes, and stroke.[20] They are, quite frankly, the worst type of fat you can eat, so much so that several countries and some regions of the U.S. have passed laws to restrict them.

Many people don't realize that there are two types of trans fats: the naturally occurring kind, which certain animals produce in their guts, and the artificial kind, which have a long history of use in commercially processed foods.[21] Most of us won't be able to remove trans fats from our diets entirely, because they are found in basic staples like meat and dairy. A small amount of this kind of trans fat is generally considered okay. It's the artificial kind, mostly found in UPFs, that we want to watch out for more, often listed on food packaging as "partially hydrogenated oil."

Trans fats have long been used in processed foods, in part because we didn't always know how bad they were for us. It's one of the main reasons why margarine has such a complicated past. During the latter half of the 20th century, margarine was touted as a healthier alternative to butter or lard, both of which contain saturated fats. That was before researchers discovered in the 1990s that trans fats were worse.

Experts recommend limiting trans fats, which is why today's margarines have largely been reformulated to avoid them. Whether today's versions are better than butter really depends on which one you choose. Butter, on the other hand, is generally okay in moderation and can be a delicious choice for the occasional baked good, for example. For everyday use, however, a better option than either of these would be a heart-healthy fat like olive oil.

Processed foods

These are foods from one of the previous two categories to which things like salt, sugar, oil, or other minimal ingredients have been added. These foods typically have just a few basic ingredients and are generally fine when consumed as one part of an overall healthy eating pattern.

Examples include:

Fresh breads, tortillas, flatbreads, and rolls

Fresh cheeses

Canned and bottled veggies and fruits with the addition of oil, salt, sugar and/or preservatives

Canned and bottled veggies or legumes preserved in brine or vinegar

Canned fish

Salted, smoked, cured, and dried fish and meats like beef jerky and smoked salmon

Salted and/or flavored nuts and seeds

Ultraprocessed foods

This is the category we are most concerned with. These are the kind of highly processed foods we described earlier, which are typically ready to eat, filled with artificial ingredients (colors, flavorings, and preservatives), and tend to be designed to induce cravings and overeating rather than nourish you.

Examples include:

Packaged snacks

Packaged cookies and crackers

Most breakfast cereals and energy bars

Many frozen desserts

Candy

Soda and sports drinks

Juices with sugar and other additives

Most premade, packaged and frozen meals

Packaged breads, tortillas, flatbreads, and rolls

Margarine

Most bottled condiments and sauces

Flavored or sweetened yogurts, milks, and milk substitutes

The NOVA Classification System can be a handy tool, but it has been faulted for leaving some things open to interpretation. A good example is yogurt. In its purest form, it is a NOVA Category 1 food containing nothing more than milk with certain cultures introduced to ferment it, turning it into yogurt. When you go to the dairy case of your grocery store, however, the definition of *yogurt* extends far beyond that. In fact, you will find an overwhelming array of options. Sitting right next to plain yogurt are flavored options that contain things like fruit concentrate, sugar, pectin, tapioca starch, guar gum, locust bean gum, natural or artificial flavors, and coloring. With some or all of these additions, a Category 1 food quickly becomes a Category 4 UPF.

Then there are the things that, strictly speaking, are processed, but that we believe are healthy. Plant-based milk substitutes, for example, are obviously processed to go from the nuts (like almonds), seeds (like flax), or grains (like oats) that we are familiar with to the cartons of liquid we find at the grocery store. And yet, we both consume them regularly. That's because they are still rather simple products with nothing much added beyond water—as long as you choose unsweetened, unflavored, and nothing-added options, of course.

More potential sources of confusion might come in the form of protein and other supplement powders. These powders are quite clearly highly processed ingredients that are classified as supplements, not food. And yet, you may have noticed that some of our Smoothie with Benefits recipes include protein powder in the ingredient list. That's largely because these kinds of products are generally made with health in mind, not to induce or satisfy cravings. We also believe they can be an effective cheat for people who are closely monitoring their protein levels, like athletes, or those who want a shortcut in the mornings when making their smoothies. We love natural proteins, of course, and believe they taste better most of the time. But protein powders can be a fine substitute if they work for you, especially if they are going to make it more likely that you will make that smoothie regularly and consume more nutrient-rich foods like fruits and veggies in the process. Even still, it is best to check labels, as not all protein powders are the same and some come with fillers and sweeteners that you just don't need. (Check out our Resources section for more information on choosing a protein powder.)

We include examples like these to illustrate how the lines can sometimes blur. It helps if you take the NOVA Classification System as a set of guidelines rather than hard-and-fast rules. Still, it can be a useful tool that works in many cases to help you look more closely at what you eat and make more informed choices.

It's the *ultra*processed foods that we want to really look at more closely, not foods that have only been processed for the sake of convenience (think nuts that have been shelled, olives that have been pitted, veggies that have been washed or cut) or for preservation (ingredients that have been frozen, dried, canned, pickled, or fermented without unwanted additives). Or even foods that have been processed with health in mind, like protein powders.

Once you learn to identify UPFs, then we can start looking at ways to easily, and without sacrificing flavor or enjoyment, move the scale from more processed to less processed options more often.

What's on Your Plate?

Over the next few days, make a point of noticing what you choose to consume. Better yet, write it down, if possible.

- Take a few minutes before each meal or snack to notice what you are about to eat. If you cooked it yourself, then note the ingredients used. If you bought it premade, then consult the package label. If it's a take-out or restaurant meal, then do your best to guess the main ingredients. Note: if you are starting your day with a Smoothie with Benefits for breakfast, then there's no need to do this for breakfast. Everything in our smoothie recipes counts as food as healthy fuel!

- As you write down what you eat, notice and mark any UPFs that you consume. It may be that the entire meal is a UPF, like a microwave dinner, or just different components, like a jarred sauce, salad dressing, packaged dessert, or snack.

- Do *not* use this list as a reason to chastise yourself for what you have eaten. Instead, use it to look for opportunities where you might be able to make healthier choices using the strategies in the rest of this chapter.

Strategy 1: Shop with Your Blender in Mind

Once you have a better idea of how much territory UPFs occupy on your plate, how do you begin to make a shift toward more as-nature-intended foods? It all starts at the grocery store, which, with all its various options, can be an overwhelming place for many of us.

A note for those of you don't cook and whose meals are mostly take-out or from restaurants: We *are* going to ask you to start going to the grocery store, at least once in a while. You will need to do this anyway—or get a CSA or grocery delivery service—to get the ingredients you need for your morning smoothies. While you are there, we hope you will shop for more than just smoothie items, because making meals yourself gives you greater control of just how healthy your food is—just how tasty and satisfying it is too! We will talk more about this subject in Chapter 6 and even teach you some simple cooking techniques, but for now, just remember our advice is to start from where you are and build from there.

To manage the overwhelming array of choices at your typical grocery store, one of the simplest strategies is to shop with your blender in mind. If you don't feel like sorting through the NOVA system or you are short on time, this strategy can work pretty well because it automatically shifts your focus toward more of the kinds of foods that provide optimal fuel for your body. That's because people are not generally inclined to throw UPFs into a blender. When we think about smoothies, blended sauces, or soups, what we think of first is usually fresh or frozen produce, nuts and seeds, canned items like tomatoes or chickpeas, maybe some minimally processed (but still plenty healthy!) options like yogurt, broths, or plant-based milks. Real, as-nature-intended food is what naturally goes into a blender, and you can use that fact to your advantage when figuring out what to buy.

Shopping with your blender in mind doesn't mean you will be drinking all your meals. In fact, if you scan our Blends with Benefits recipes in Chapter 7, you may even be able to expand your definition of what works in a blender. It's not limited to stuff in the produce aisle but also includes meat and eggs (try our **Blender Chicken Salad Spread** or **Egg-Cellent Egg Salad Spread** on page 227) and whole grains and legumes (see our **Red Lentil Wraps** or **Oat Naan** recipes on pages 223 and 225). In fact, we have a whole category of Unexpected Blender Recipes, and even these feature healthy, as-nature-intended ingredients.

Another way to look at this is that we are asking you to **prioritize "nonlabel foods"**—meaning there are no labels listing the ingredients or nutritional information. This basic rule of thumb works because, in the U.S., where food labeling is overseen by the Food and Drug Administration (FDA), such labels are required only on prepared foods that have more than one ingredient.[22] If the food you are contemplating buying is straightforward enough that it doesn't need a label to tell you what's in it—like broccoli, cherries, chicken, or scallops—then it is food as nature intended.

FuelUp

This is where you can start. Fill up your cart with as many blender-ready, nonlabel foods as you want. That means you can begin in the produce aisle or the produce section of the frozen-food aisle, move on to proteins—meat, fish, eggs—and then go from there.

Strategy 2: Uplevel Your Basics

Upleveling is a strategy we are going to use throughout this book, which basically means to find ways to add healthy nutrients to what you are already eating.

In terms of choosing more as-nature-intended foods over UPFs, this can mean two things. First, you can consult package labels to look for **healthier versions of the staples you use again and again**. Wherever possible, ask yourself: Is there a version of this that is affordable and that I will still enjoy but is less processed or a bit healthier in some way?

Maybe you often grab strawberry yogurt for a quick snack, for example, but you notice your preferred brand has added sugar and fillers. Why not buy the plain version and add fresh or frozen strawberries yourself? The same idea works with oatmeal. Buy plain oats and add your own toppings rather than choosing the instant, flavored versions. When it comes to packaged foods like sauces, condiments, and salad dressings, look for options that have fewer ingredients, little or no added sugars, and few, if any, artificial or unrecognizable ingredients. Reading labels can feel like a bit of a hassle, but remember, once you have found something that works, then you can buy that same product again and again without giving it a second thought.

Another way to uplevel your basics is to keep the processed food options you already like and **look for ways to add nutrition**. For example, we are often told that brown rice is better for you than white rice. It's less processed and, as a result, has more essential fiber (a subject we will talk more about in the next chapter). Quinoa or farro are also great whole-grain options that we recommend, which can often be used in place of rice. But if you prefer white rice, then choose white rice—especially if *not* choosing it is going to make you enjoy your food less. And don't feel bad about it! After all, lots of cultures from Mexico to Japan have been using white rice for generations in their cooking.

We love sushi, for example, and even though a lot of American sushi restaurants offer a brown-rice option these days, there are plenty of people who like traditional white-rice versions better.

What you can do instead is think about how you can add nutrition to the processed foods you do choose. **Uplevel** a white-rice-and-chicken dish by adding a nutrient-rich sauce or a condiment that can be made fresh in your blender in just a few minutes. An easy, tomato-based salsa with jalapeño, onion, and cilantro offers a range of essential nutrients, including vitamin K, vitamin B_6, potassium, manganese, and a generous dose of vitamin C. It also has fiber! So, you are adding back some of the fiber that was lost when brown rice was milled to remove its bran layer and turn it into white rice.

The same strategy works with packaged foods like sauces or soups. We would love it if you made your own tomato soup from scratch, for example, using only as-nature-intended ingredients. But if there's a canned soup that's a family favorite, or just a favorite convenience after a long day (the reality is that the famed Campbell's tomato soup alone sells 85 million cans a year in the U.S.[23]), think about it as the perfect vehicle for tossing in a handful of spinach, pinches of fresh or dried herbs, and/or a package of frozen mixed veggies—all of which can turn this pantry staple into healthier fuel for your body. If you don't like veggie chunks in your tomato soup, or if someone in your house won't eat it if he sees something green floating in it, then use your blender to puree your vegetable additions with a cupful of the soup. Your picky eater will hardly notice the difference!

If you do these kinds of simple upgrades with enough items in your fridge and pantry, it can make a real difference over time. Remember, the goal here is to consume *fewer* UPFs. If you are like most people, whose diet consists of more than 50 percent UPFs, then you will likely find lots of opportunities to uplevel by either subbing in foods that are less processed or enhancing the ones you can't live without.

Try our Did Someone Say Salsa? (page 200) or Mighty Mango Salsa (page 200) recipes for delicious homemade condiments that add flavor *and* nutrition to your dishes.

Strategy 3: DIY Processing

One of our favorite strategies for cutting back on ultraprocessed foods is to do the "processing" ourselves at home. It allows us to have more control over the ingredients we use so that we can choose to leave out or minimize the less optimal stuff—like added sugars, excess fat and salt, additives, and preservatives. It also gives us a chance to make more nutrient-dense versions of our favorite things. And yummier versions that are more tailored to our tastes! Your blender, of course, is the perfect tool for this.

DIY processing works well for all sorts of things. Sauces, marinades, condiments, dressings, snacks, and even desserts can often be made healthier when you make them yourself. For example, Dr. Dana used to have a coveted steak sauce brand that she returned to again and again. Made by a well-known restaurant that started bottling their sauce only after customers begged them to, Dr. Dana used it for years before she thought to look at the label. High on the ingredient list was sugar, followed by high-fructose corn syrup, followed by corn syrup, followed a bit lower down by molasses. That's four different kinds of sugar! Also included were "natural flavors" and coloring. She couldn't believe it. A little bit of one kind of sugar was one thing, but this seemed like overkill. And so unnecessary. She was convinced the flavor she loved could be achieved without all the extras, so she set out to make her own version at home. After some experimentation, she and a friend came up with a recipe that combines tomato paste, vinegar, horseradish, onion, garlic, lemon, and just a little maple syrup. It's not only healthier, but she thinks it tastes better too. (You will find the recipe at the end of this chapter so you can try it for yourself!)

Many of our Blends with Benefits recipes in Chapter 7 will help you do this, and it's often not as time-consuming as you might think. For our delicious **Enhanced Stir-Fry Sauce** (page 184), you need just five common ingredients, it can be whipped up in a couple of minutes, and it's much healthier than bottled versions. Our **Beyond Bean Dip** (page 201) is much tastier (in our opinion) than what you find in jars at the supermarket and requires no cooking at all—just toss the ingredients in your blender and hit the button. We ask only that you try a few of these and see how much better they can be—not just for your body, but for your taste buds as well.

3 Ways to Uplevel Your Salad Dressing

The strategies we just covered work for all sorts of different foods. We are providing you with a couple of examples here to help you think through what will work for you and for the people you cook and eat with. Consider the following options when it comes to salad dressings, choose what works best for you today, and don't sweat it if you don't always choose the health*iest* option. Health*ier* is often good enough.

Healthy-Enough Option: Salad! with Store-bought Dressing: Look, even if you're using a store-bought salad dressing that has some less-than-optimal ingredients, you are still eating salad, which is almost surely composed mostly, if not entirely, of nonlabel ingredients. For many of us, that counts as a win. Where possible, consider checking the label on your bottled salad dressing and opting for healthier versions with less fat and little or no sugars or additives, even if you just rotate it in once in a while.

Health*ier* Option: Oil and Vinegar: It's an old Italian staple to drizzle a little olive oil and balsamic vinegar on a salad. Add a dash of salt and pepper, and you're good to go. It's the simplest dressing there is, and it's plenty healthy. If you're going to try this option, consider investing in a high-quality, fruity olive oil and a high-quality vinegar, not so much for health reasons as for the taste. If you enjoy it, you are much more likely to continue making this healthy choice.

Health*iest* Option: DIY Salad Dressing: We love creating dressings that add an extra nutritional punch to salads and veggies, and they really aren't difficult to make. They rarely require cooking and can often be whipped up in your blender in just a few minutes. Experiment and create your own concoctions or try our **Enhanced Ranch Dressing** or other dressing recipes on page 188.

3 Ways to Uplevel Your Red Sauce

Many of us keep jars of pasta sauce in the pantry for quick and easy meals. There's nothing wrong with that. And yet, it still may provide an opportunity to uplevel your meal!

Healthy-Enough Option: Souped-Up Sauce: If your preferred jarred red sauce brand includes things like added sugar or preservatives but it's still the best option for you for reasons of cost, accessibility, or even just because you or your family don't like anything else, then consider doctoring it up with added nutrients. Throw in some olives or capers, fresh or dried herbs, or extra veggies. Consider pureeing those veggies if seeing them floating in the sauce turns you off. This will make for a more nutrient-dense meal.

Health_ier_ Option: High-Quality Jarred Marinara Sauce: Healthier options can be found at the grocery store if you look for them. If you read labels, you will find there are a number of jarred sauce brands on the market with minimal processing and just a few simple ingredients like tomatoes, onion, olive oil, garlic, herbs, and salt and pepper. That's it. No fillers. No extras. Nothing we wouldn't include if we were making a marinara ourselves. Unfortunately, options like these can be a bit more expensive, so that's something to consider.

Health_iest_ Option: DIY Pasta Sauce: Dr. Dana believes that even the best jarred sauces never taste as good as freshly made, which is why she prefers her quick recipe for what she calls her "homestyle tomato sauce." It uses only as-nature-intended ingredients and couldn't be easier: Sauté sliced garlic in a good amount of olive oil in a large skillet until lightly browned. Add chopped fresh tomatoes of any kind; even cherry or grape tomatoes will do, or canned diced tomatoes if that's what you have on hand. (This is a great way to use up fresh tomatoes that are starting to wrinkle!) Toss in some salt and maybe a little dried oregano if you have it. Let the mixture cook down for about 20 to 30 minutes, then toss in your pasta. The key is to use good olive oil to enhance the flavor. Dr. Dana insists it's one of her favorite meals. She dares you to go back to jarred sauce after trying it!

So-Called Healthy Food Claims: "Light" and "Natural" and "Organic," Oh My

We need to include a word here on some of the different food-labeling terms, because when you are evaluating your food choices, you may find that they can be difficult to understand to the point of downright dizzying. Research suggests that shoppers often consider a food better for them if they see a "health" claim on its packaging,[24] even though these claims don't always equate to health. In fact, one study found that some food companies take advantage of this perception by using healthy-sounding labels on foods that really aren't very healthy. Nearly half (48 percent) of the foods studied with these kinds of labels were actually not so healthy after all, typically because they were high in saturated fat, salt, and/or sugar.[25]

Some of the most confounding terms include:

Light: This simply means the product is a reduced-calorie and/or reduced-fat version of the original, like a light mayonnaise or a light Caesar dressing. However, *lower* isn't the same as being *low* in fat or calories. Also, manufacturers often compensate for lost fat, which lends flavor, with something else, like sugar. When you see this term, it's best to look closely at the ingredients and nutritional information before you buy.

Multigrain: This term tends to signal "healthiness" to shoppers, and that can be true. The thing to understand, however, is that it simply means that more than one grain is included. All those grains may be refined, and, if they are, they have likely lost nutrients, like fiber, during processing. Products labeled *whole grain*—regardless of whether it's one grain or multiple grains—are generally healthier options.

Natural: Sadly, some common packaging terms, like *natural*, don't mean much at all. For example, the snack-food giant Frito Lay calls some of their cheese puffs "Natural Cheetos." Cheetos are obviously a UPF and not what most reasonable people would think of as natural. So-called natural choices are readily available throughout the supermarket, some good, some less so, but the term doesn't have an official definition. (At one point, the government did try to come up with one but then abandoned course.)[26] Because its definition is so squishy, the term is best ignored.

Organic: Organics are an even more nuanced case. To many consumers, *organic* means healthier, and unlike the term *natural*, *organic* does have an official definition. According to the USDA, which regulates the use of the word on food packaging: "Organic is a labeling term that indicates that the food or other agricultural product has been produced through approved methods. These methods integrate cultural, biological, and mechanical practices that foster cycling of resources, promote ecological balance, and conserve biodiversity."[27]

Does that clear things up for you? We didn't think so. Confusion can breed misinformation, such as the popular notion that organic farming doesn't use pesticides. Not true. While conventional pesticides and synthetic fertilizers are not allowed, there is a list of pesticides that are approved for organic farming, including some synthetic pesticides.

A systematic review of dozens of studies related to the health benefits of organic versus conventional food found that "the current evidence base does not allow a definitive statement on the health benefits of organic dietary intake."[28] There have been individual studies linking a higher intake of organics with a lower risk of certain negative health outcomes, but a link is not the same as saying that eating organics *causes* health benefits. It would be nice if eating well meant simply sticking to foods with the organic label, but unfortunately, more research is needed before anyone can say definitively whether it's worth it.

Does this mean you shouldn't choose organics? Not necessarily. We often choose them ourselves and think it's fine to shop according to your values. However, you don't need to feel like you've done something wrong if you don't or can't. While we personally love a good organic farmer's market, we are also aware that there are cost and accessibility factors involved in this choice that don't suit everyone. The truth of the matter is that buying organic is less important from a nutritional perspective than simply eating more real, as-nature-intended foods. That means that, sure, fresh, organic peas are a great option. But so are fresh, nonorganic peas, or the frozen kind (whether organic or not), which are often cheaper and won't spoil as quickly. The point is to just eat more peas (and other as-nature-intended foods)!

What it comes down to is this: don't get caught up in labels if it's going to stress you out, cost too much, or get in the way of enjoying what you eat. One of the best ways to avoid the hassle of reading and trying to understand those package labels is to avoid, as much as possible, the foods that require them, which is why we suggested earlier that you start your shopping by filling your cart with as-nature-intended options or what we call nonlabel foods. Then there will be fewer things that require a closer look.

If you can and want to choose foods with certain labels, like organics, then please do. If you can't or don't want to, then just make sure to clean your ingredients well to remove any residue. But you will want to clean your produce anyway—even organics can have dirt, bacteria, pests, and pesticide residue—so it's not even an extra step. (Don't forget about the Best Way to Clean Your Produce directions we provided in Chapter 1.) When it comes to as-nature-intended foods, just buy what you like and what works for you. And then eat it!

More Cheats to Try

Following are a few additional tips that can make minimizing UPFs and maximizing foods as nature intended that much easier and more enjoyable.

Grow Something! Colin is lucky enough to have an edible garden at his home, which he makes use of daily. His morning Smoothie with Benefits typically includes greens from his garden—kales, Swiss chard, and/or spinach leaves—and whatever else is in season, which could be beets with their leaves, carrots with their tops, or all sorts of other options. He also likes to visit the garden when he needs a snack, which could be Fuji apples one day or blackberries another. It makes it that much easier to make healthy choices when such an inspiring array of nature's bounty is so accessible to him!

Of course, we don't all have the space or time for a garden of that scale, but there are simpler ways to try out your green thumb. A window box of herbs is a great place to start. Microgreens and sprouts can be grown on your kitchen counter without taking up a lot of space. The next time you buy scallions, cut off the root ends and place them in a jar of fresh water on your windowsill. Change the water weekly, and snip off the tops when you're ready to use them. The point is that when you have fresh, as-nature-intended food around, you will be that much more inspired to make use of it!

Let Your Grocer "Process" Food for You. Rotisserie chicken. Freshly made soups and salads. A good grocery store, butcher, or fish market can be your best friend when you are trying to eat more real food but are short on time or energy. A couple of notes: this can be more expensive, so it may be a cheat you use only occasionally, and it's best to check labels before you buy. But if the ingredient list includes the same things you would use yourself if you made it, then go for it. As the molecular biologist and nutritionist Marion Nestle put it, "If you can make it in your home kitchen, it's not ultra-processed because ultra-processing requires ingredients that you don't have and machinery that you don't have."[29] This is also an opportunity for upleveling: add veggies, herbs, spices, nuts, seeds—whatever sounds good to enhance both the nutrients and flavor of what you bought.

Whole Foods Can Mean the Whole Food. Here's a great tip for upleveling your nutrients and doing less work at the same time: when it comes to plants, consume more parts of your food. That means leaves, skins, stalks, seeds—the stuff that so often ends up in the trash. Much of what we throw out is actually edible and may even be highly nutritious.

Take skins, for example. Why would anyone choose to peel an apple or a tomato or even a potato? People do it, and you will find lots of recipes that suggest it. Chefs will generally tell you it's for the sake of appearance and texture, but it's certainly not a matter of nutrition (or taste, if you ask us). Remember the old adage that an apple a day keeps the doctor away? Well, it should specify that an *unpeeled* apple keeps the doctor away, because the peel is where you will find the bulk of the beneficial antioxidants. Beet greens, too, are often overlooked, but they are highly nutritious, rich in calcium, iron, vitamin K, and B vitamins. Ginger skin contains protective phytonutrients. Broccoli leaves, strawberry leaves, and carrot tops (not to mention the peels . . . why waste time peeling?), among many other options, all have nutritional benefits that we could be taking advantage of, with the added benefit that doing so cuts down on food waste (good for the environment) as well as prep and cleanup time (good for us!).

Blending makes this especially easy. Making a smoothie? Throw in whole strawberries, tops and all, or ginger with its peel. Celery with its leaves. Carrots washed but unpeeled. Not just the red part of the watermelon, but also the white—which has a higher concentration of fiber and potassium.[30] You will lose none of the flavor (you won't even notice the difference), and you will gain nutrients. Leaves from veggies like broccoli, beets, and cauliflower can be blended into a sauce. Carrot tops make a great base or addition to pesto, chimichurri, or hummus. Once you get used to looking at your produce differently, there are numerous possibilities to try.

Of course, not everything is edible. Things like peach pits, apricot pits, apple seeds, and cherimoya seeds can be toxic and should be discarded. Others, like date pits, are edible but too hard to process in a blender without roasting them first. If in doubt, do a quick Google search to find out, but chances are, the "do not eat" list is a lot shorter than you think.

Recipe to Try Today! A Health*ier* Condiment That Is Fun to Make and Delicious to Eat

Made largely from fresh or minimally processed ingredients, Dr. Dana's favorite steak sauce recipe still has a hint of sweetness in the form of maple syrup but has far less sugar than most bottled versions. Maple syrup is also a bit lower on the glycemic index—a scale that indicates how quickly and how high your blood sugar rises after ingesting a carb-rich food—than table sugar, and it has the added benefit of being loaded with antioxidants and minerals. Just make sure that what you use comes from real maple trees.

SUPERB STEAK SAUCE

Makes about 6 servings

1 cup diced yellow onion
2 garlic cloves
Juice of 1 lemon
¼ cup maple syrup
2 tablespoons tomato paste
1 tablespoon white vinegar
1 tablespoon Worcestershire sauce
1 to 2 teaspoons prepared horseradish
¼ cup water

Sauté the onions and garlic in a pot for a few minutes, until tender.

Add the remaining ingredients. Simmer the mixture on low heat for about 20 minutes, whisking occasionally until the sauce thickens.

Cool the ingredients. Add them to the blender and blend until smooth.

Pour the sauce into a storage container. Keep it in the refrigerator and enjoy for up to 1 month.

Cheat Sheet

3 Ways to Consume More Foods as Nature Intended . . . Right Away!

1. **Shop with Your Blender in Mind**
   At the grocery store, think about what works best in your blender. This will help you prioritize nonlabel foods and less processed items, because that's what works best in a blender. Fruits, veggies, nuts, seeds, whole grains, legumes, unprocessed meats, and fish are all great choices. And remember: a greater balance of these versus ultraprocessed foods is what you are aiming for.

2. **Uplevel Your Basics**
   When buying packaged or processed foods, check the label and look for options with fewer and more straightforward ingredients and with few (or no) additives where possible. And if that doesn't work, stick with your standbys and find ways to add nutrients.

3. **DIY Processed Food**
   Where possible, try making your own versions of common processed foods at home using a higher proportion of natural and nutritious ingredients—a cheat that is not as time-consuming as it may sound when you use your blender. Check our recipe chapter for ideas on how to do this for everything from sauces and dressings to snacks and desserts.

CHAPTER 3

Variety Variety Variety

Fuel Up Habit #3

Eat more kinds, more colors, and just more plants!

For your next Fuel Up Habit, we are going to focus not just on eating more real foods but on eating a greater variety of those foods, especially plants.

Once again, this advice is meant to be simple, straightforward, and, most of all, doable. The reasoning behind it has to do with the fact that, in order to thrive, our bodies need to be provided with a broad spectrum of nutrients. There are your basic macronutrients (protein, carbs, and fats), a long list of micronutrients (vitamins and minerals), and an even longer list of phytonutrients (compounds found in plants). How can we make sure we are getting all the right stuff? And that we are getting the right stuff in the right amounts?

We're not going to lie to you: determining exactly how much of each nutrient you are consuming is nearly impossible unless you have access to a lab and the time and resources needed to test the nutrient content of every single thing you eat. There are plenty of calorie counters out there, where you plug in what you eat and they tell you roughly how many calories you have consumed, but that's a woefully inadequate measure of health. Most packaged foods come with Nutrition Facts labels that include Daily Value (DV) percentages, but it's debatable whether those are even useful. For one thing, they aren't exhaustive. Food companies are required only to list a few select micronutrients (though some may choose to list more) and no phytonutrients at all.[1] Plus, not everything comes with a label.

Even if we could get complete nutrition info on all the things we eat, would any of us really have the time or the wherewithal to do all that math? The label on a can of chickpeas, for example, might tell you that its contents have 12 percent of your recommended daily intake of protein per serving, 10 percent of your RDI of iron, and 4 percent of your calcium RDI. Sounds straightforward enough, but if you then blend those chickpeas with tahini, garlic, and lemon juice, top that with a little olive oil and parsley, and eat the mixture with cucumber slices and pita bread, how much of these nutrients would you be getting exactly? And that's just a basic hummus recipe. Imagine the estimations and calculations that would go into figuring out a complete nutritional profile for a complex meal, let alone a whole day's worth of eating. Or a week's. It's enough to make your head spin.

To be fully fueled, having a varied diet is a *realistic* way to cover your bases without all the head-spinning. Your body needs a wide variety of nutrients in different forms and amounts, so it makes sense to consume a wide variety of foods that are quality sources of those nutrients. That means more foods as nature intended, as we talked about in the last chapter, and plants in particular. That's because over and over again, it has been shown that plants are essential to good health. We will cover some of the research in the coming pages, but to cite just one example, a 2023 cohort study of more than 125,000 participants found that a healthy, plant-based diet was associated with a lower risk not just of certain conditions like cardiovascular disease and cancer, but also of overall mortality.[2]

It's for this reason that, later in this chapter, we are going to ask you to look a little more closely at what you are eating and then try what we call a **plant-positive diet**, which simply means starting from wherever you are already in terms of your plant consumption and then find ways to add more, both in terms of variety and volume. It's important to understand, however, that "plant-positive" doesn't mean plant-only. You don't have to be a vegetarian or vegan to be healthy (although you can if you choose). Plant-adding is for everyone. No matter what diet you follow, or if you follow no particular diet at all, you can benefit from choosing more plants more often.

We are even going to give you a target number to shoot for: 30 plants per week! That may sound like a lot right now, but we think you'll find that blending makes it a whole lot easier. Besides, you may not realize just how many of the things you are already eating count as plants. We are not just talking about fruits and vegetables here, but also herbs, spices, nuts, seeds, whole grains, legumes—even coffee and cocoa beans (so, chocolate counts!)—which means there are plenty of options to choose from. But, before you start adding plants, we are going to take a closer look at just how much you can gain if you do.

Case Study: Stephanie and Adam

Stephanie and Adam were starting from different places when they began blending regularly. "I do pretty well with my health and nutrition," Stephanie said. She was a regular tennis player who already made a point of doing her best to eat well even though, as a mom to two active kids ages 10 and 12, she was always on the go.

Adam, on the other hand, had always been a steak-and-potatoes guy. When Stephanie first met him, she would laugh about the "salads" he ate. "I think you have a little bit of iceberg in there with your ranch dressing," she liked to say to him.

Adam admitted that changing some of his eating habits was a little tough at first, but it was still "a lot easier" to throw the plants he had been missing into a blender rather than having a big side dish of veggies at dinner. It just worked better for him than force-feeding himself a bowl of spinach, and he was able to consume more plants than ever before.

Stephanie, on the other hand, started blending in large part because she knew that if she did it, "my husband will have to do it." But she found that she benefited too. Even though she was already eating well, she was able to add even more plants to her daily diet by tossing them into her blends. "You don't taste them, so it's like, why not?" she explained. "Why not throw that extra stuff in there and know that you're doing that much more good for your body?"

After eating a greater amount and variety of plants every day for several weeks, both Stephanie and Adam noticed they were feeling better. They kept up their new healthy eating habits, not only because of how it made them feel, but also to set an example for their kids. They had always told the kids that they needed to eat their fruits and vegetables, but, as Adam admitted, they didn't always practice what they preached.

Now the kids saw their parents actually enjoying fruits and veggies every day, and they got excited about it. "They were constantly asking before school, 'Well, if you're having a shake, can I have a shake?' And after school, 'Well, if you're having an afternoon blend, can I have an afternoon blend?'" Stephanie said. The whole family started washing, cutting, blending, and drinking their smoothies together in the mornings, which was a really great way to start the day.

"It really helped bond our family," Stephanie said. Which may be the best reason of all!

Maximize Your Micronutrients

One of the ways that a varied diet will help you become fully fueled is by maximizing your intake of micronutrients, which are all those vitamins and minerals, from *vitamin A* to *zinc*, that our bodies need but (in most cases) can't make on their own, so they have to be obtained through food. As opposed to macronutrients, which our bodies require in large quantities, we need only small amounts of micronutrients (hence the *micro* part of the word), but that doesn't make them unimportant.

The essential mineral potassium, for example—which is found in foods like apricots, raisins, avocados, bananas, beans, and legumes—can be found in all the tissues in the body and is required for proper cellular function. And yet, surveys show that Americans consistently consume less than the recommended amounts.[3] Perhaps not surprisingly, then, low potassium intake can result in conditions that are fairly common, like kidney stones and high blood pressure. A true deficiency can result in something called *hypokalemia*, symptoms of which include everything from fatigue and muscle weakness to glucose intolerance, respiratory issues, and arrhythmia. Severe cases can even be life-threatening. Potassium is also an electrolyte, which plays a role in keeping the body hydrated (a subject we will cover in detail in Chapter 4).

Vitamin E, on the other hand, is mostly found in an entirely different set of foods from the ones that feature potassium—particularly nuts, seeds, vegetable oils, and leafy greens like spinach and broccoli—as well as fortified products like cereals, milk, and milk substitutes. As a fat-soluble antioxidant, this vitamin plays a vital role in protecting us from unstable chemicals called *free radicals*, which can damage cells and may contribute to the development of diseases like cancer and heart disease.[4] While outright deficiencies are rare in the U.S., nutrition surveys suggest that many of us still may not be getting optimal amounts.[5, 6]

There are around 30 different micronutrients that our bodies need on a regular basis to be fully fueled. Vitamin B_{12} (fish, meat, dairy), aka *cobalamin*, is one of eight in the family of B vitamins and helps convert food into energy. Calcium (seeds, dairy, fish with edible bones like sardines) is needed for strong bones and muscle function. Vitamin C (citrus, berries, peppers) helps keep your immune system functioning properly. We could keep going, but you get the idea. All micronutrients play a vital role in our health and well-being, and each one is present at different levels in different foods.

As important as micronutrients are, most of us probably couldn't list them all, let alone describe their crucial functions. In fact, we probably don't think much about them at all unless our doctor tells us that we have some sort of deficiency. And that can happen. In fact, the 2020–2025 *Dietary Guidelines for Americans* report identifies several nutrients to pay particular attention to: "Calcium, potassium, dietary fiber, and vitamin D are considered dietary components of public health concern for the general U.S. population."[7]

We strongly recommend that you get annual blood tests to flag such things where possible, but that alone is not enough to ensure you are fully fueled. It can take a while for deficiencies to show up in your bloodwork, and many micronutrients, like vitamin E, aren't routinely tested for. What's more, even if you don't have a clinical deficiency, your intake could still be lower than optimal levels for your health and well-being—something we call a "nutritional shortfall."

It's for all these reasons and more that a varied diet of nutrient-rich foods is so important. As you can tell by our examples, different foods provide different benefits, so casting a wide nutritional net is the most practical way to ensure you are getting everything you need.

Micronutrient Maximizers: Salad Shooters

In the first chapter, we briefly introduced you to our Salad Shooters, which are three-gulp smoothies packed with greens and other nutrient-rich ingredients that we sometimes use as a pregaming strategy—a quick way to provide our bodies with a dose of nutrients and hydration before heading out on the town.

But that's not all that Salad Shooters are good for. They are also a great way to get your leafy greens. Even if you don't like green things like spinach, arugula, parsley, kale, and other lettuces, it's worth trying to find a way to consume them that you will actually enjoy. That's because they have *soooo* many health benefits. When researchers at the Centers for Disease Control (CDC) set out to rank the nutrient density of a wide variety of vegetables and fruits, they found that 17 of the top 20 foods were greens, which typically feature a treasure trove of micronutrients including B vitamins, vitamin C, calcium, vitamin E, iron, vitamin K, magnesium, and potassium.[8] It's no wonder then that these nutrient powerhouses are linked to a reduced risk of chronic diseases like diabetes, heart disease, certain cancers, and more. One recent study even found that daily greens may slow cognitive decline and help preserve your memory.[9]

Our Smoothies with Benefits can be a great way to add greens, and our Salad Shooters are another. Dr. Dana likes to recommend that you have either a salad or a Salad Shooter as an amuse-bouche before dinner. It's a way to wake up your palate and ensure you get some quality nutrients no matter what's on the menu for dinner. It also means that you get your fiber first (fiber being an important topic that we will cover later in this chapter). Finally, there is some evidence to suggest that eating veggies and proteins before carbs can lead to less elevated glucose levels.[10] It's a fact that more than one-third of American adults have prediabetes and another 11 percent have overt diabetes, and this may be a useful tip to help some people stabilize blood sugar.[11]

Another benefit of our Salad Shooters is that they all contain a healthy fat in the form of olive oil. Vitamins come in two types: water soluble and fat soluble; the latter being ones that get absorbed by our bodies along with the fats in food. The excess then gets stored in fat tissue and the liver, where it remains for a period of time, waiting to be used, which is a handy way that our remarkable bodies do their best to make sure we have what we need even if we're not consuming the nutrient every day. Our Salad Shooters contain olive oil to enable absorption of fat-soluble vitamins, which include vitamins A, D, E, and K. It's worth noting that only excess fat-soluble vitamins get stored in the body, not excess water-soluble ones, which get eliminated when you urinate. As a result, water-soluble vitamins—vitamin C and the family of B vitamins—need to be consumed more regularly to give the body what it needs.

Shoot Your Salad Leftovers!

If you're someone who enjoys salad, the Salad Shooter concept is a great cheat for using up leftovers. Because dressed greens don't keep very well and instead end up all limp and soggy, we suggest you blend them to make your own salad shooter. This may sound a little strange at first, but you will be surprised by how good it can taste. We recently tried it with a leftover salad of mixed greens, toasted pecans, pomegranate seeds, goat cheese, and a champagne vinaigrette. It was delicious! If your salad has been dressed with a vinegar-based dressing, the blend will typically taste like a shrub, which is a kind of vinegar-based drink that's enjoyed throughout the world. It was even popular in colonial America and has made a resurgence in recent years.

If your leftover salad shooter doesn't taste so great, then toss it. That's probably what you would have done anyway with those soggy greens, so no loss. But you might just find that it's a delicious way to create a quick, nutrient-rich snack *and* avoid food waste at the same time. So why not give it a try?

Pile on the Phytonutrients

The prefix *phyto-* means "plants," so the word *phytonutrient* simply means that, unlike micronutrients—which can be found in plant and animal foods—these nutrients are found only in plants. The main category of phytonutrients that we want to talk about here is polyphenols. With names like *quercetin* (found in apples), *catechin* (green tea), *anthocyanin* (blueberries), and *kaempferol* (kale), you have probably heard about them in the news because a high polyphenol content is often the reason why something gets categorized as a superfood. (For the record, the term *superfood* has no official meaning and is as much a marketing term as anything else, but the antioxidant and anti-inflammatory power of polyphenol-containing foods is real.)

In simple terms, polyphenols are compounds synthesized by plants for a variety of reasons, like helping them to adapt to temperature variations or protect themselves against pests or fungal infections. It seems that the beneficial nature of these compounds gets passed on to us when we eat them. As a whole, a diet rich in polyphenols is associated with a reduced risk of chronic diseases, including cardiovascular disease, certain cancers, neurodegenerative diseases, and type 2 diabetes.[12, 13] There's also evidence that such a diet contributes to a healthy gut and metabolism and may even improve mood and sleep disorders.[14]

While phytonutrients are not considered essential to basic functioning in the same way that macro- and micronutrients are, the new consensus in nutrition is that plants are central to disease prevention and healing. Studies are ongoing in this area, and the truth is that we don't know all the details of how or why polyphenols benefit us—just that there's strong evidence that they do.[15, 16] As the authors of one systematic review of studies related to polyphenol consumption and health outcomes put it: a polyphenol-rich dietary pattern "should be considered a valid tool for the prevention of numerous chronic diseases."[17]

There are more than 8,000 polyphenols in all, so naturally they come from a wide variety of plants and provide a wide range of benefits. Take the tomato, which is the second-most consumed vegetable in the U.S., after the humble potato and just before onions.[18] Tomatoes contain a polyphenol called lycopene, which gives them their bright-red color. Probably because of their distinct color, tomatoes, which are native to the Andes region in South America, were called "love apples" when they were first brought to England in the 16th century.[19] Coincidentally, these plants are now known to be good for our hearts. Lycopene in tomatoes has been linked to a reduced risk of heart disease and stroke.[20] Lycopene is an antioxidant—meaning it helps protect our cells from damage from free radicals—which is why tomatoes are linked to cancer prevention, particularly prostate cancer.[21] Furthermore, tomatoes contain phytonutrients known as carotenoids, which our bodies transform into vitamin A, a micronutrient essential to healthy eyes, skin, and hair. With all these benefits, it's too bad the 16th-century Britons didn't eat their tomatoes. Back then, tomato plants were largely ornamental and believed to be toxic throughout much of Europe and North America, a sad misconception that lasted in some places for hundreds of years. What a waste of a nutritious and delicious plant!

Phytonutrient Pile-On Strategy:
Add Color to Your Meals

When looking to add plants to your meals, an effective cheat is to focus on adding a wide variety of colors. This advice doesn't mean that you should avoid less colorful foods like browns and tans, which are the dominate colors among whole categories of food staples like meats and whole grains. It just means you can look for ways to be additive, upleveling those staples by adding color. A not-so-colorful chicken wrap, for example, would be greatly enhanced, nutrient- and flavor-wise, by the addition of guacamole, which could include red tomatoes, purple onions, and green avocados, jalapeños, and cilantro, plus maybe a splash of yellow lemon juice!

This advice works because different colors indicate different phytonutrients, so adding color, sometimes referred to as "eating the rainbow," helps us get a greater variety of nutrients. Many people don't realize that even different-colored varieties of the same ingredient have different nutrient profiles. You may have noticed, for example, that while most of the carrots found in a typical supermarket are orange, that isn't the only option. In fact, it's believed that wild carrots originated in the Middle East more than a thousand years ago, and, at the time, they were either purple or yellow.[22] Today you can still find such varieties, along with red and white. According to Philipp Simon, a research geneticist at the USDA, each has its own nutrient profile thanks to the different pigments: Orange carrots have beta and alpha carotene, which benefit your eyes and immune system. Purple carrots have anthocyanin and can help prevent heart disease and stroke. Yellow carrots have xanthophylls and promote eye health. Red carrots, like tomatoes, have lycopene, which has been linked to prostate cancer prevention.[23]

Some of the colors that indicate different beneficial compounds include:

Red-Orange: Beta-carotene found in cantaloupe, pumpkins, mango, and sweet potatoes.

Bright Red: Lycopene found in tomatoes, watermelon, cranberries, and red grapefruit.

Green: Chlorophyll found in broccoli, kale, spinach, parsley, celery, and sprouts.

Yellow: Zeaxanthin found in corn, yellow squash, saffron, egg yolks, and paprika.

Purple/Blue: Anthocyanin found in acai berries, blueberries, black currants, purple grapes, purple potatoes, eggplant, plums, and figs.

White: Anthoxanthin found in cauliflower, onions, potatoes, and turnips.

This is hardly an exhaustive list, and most plant foods contain more than one compound. Many green veggies, for example, often include a mix of the polyphenols sulforaphane, isothiocyanates, and indoles. Do you need to remember terms like these when you are at the grocery store deciding what to buy? Of course not. You just need to look for colors. Aim for the whole spectrum of colors if you can.

The thinking behind this, like most of the advice we offer you, is to have a simple, easy-to-remember way to approach your food choices, one that allows you to layer on the nutrients. It's an appealing way to eat, too, not to mention highly Instagrammable for those who like to snap pictures of their food. As the old saying goes, "We eat with our eyes first," and colorful foods certainly satisfy that.

Color Stars Worth Adding

These colorful fruits may be harder to find in some places, but we think they are worth hunting for because they are delicious, nutritious, *and* pretty to look at. In addition to all the different phytonutrients and micronutrients they contain, each is a significant source of fiber. Eat them on their own, add them to your smoothies, or use them to top a smoothie bowl (directions on page 176). And don't forget to snap a picture before you dig in!

- **Passion Fruit:** This tart and tangy tropical fruit boasts different-colored exteriors, but the antioxidant-rich pulp inside is typically yellow.

- **Dragon Fruit:** The bright pink, spiky bulbs of this fruit from the cactus family stand in contrast to the mild sweetness of the flesh inside, which can be either white or pink.

- **Papaya:** Also mildly sweet in flavor, the red, orange, or yellow flesh of papaya is often used in marinades because it contains an enzyme that helps tenderize meat.

- **Guava:** Common throughout Mexico and Central and South America, guava flesh is sweet with a hint of acidity and comes in a variety of colors, including pink, salmon, and red.

You may have noticed earlier in this chapter that dietary fiber was deemed a "public health concern" in the *Dietary Guidelines for Americans* report. That's because more than 90 percent of women and 97 percent of men do not get enough of it, largely due to the underconsumption of plants.[24] Despite these dismal numbers, consumer research suggests that most people are aware of fiber's importance to their health and believe they already get enough of it.[25] Clearly there's a disconnect here.

So what is fiber exactly? It's a kind of carbohydrate found in plants. There are two types, and both are important for good health:

Soluble fiber is a kind of fiber that attracts water and dissolves in it, forming a gel-like substance. As a result, it slows down digestion, which helps keep our blood sugar from spiking (a particular benefit for people with prediabetes or diabetes). It also may help to prevent heart disease. Soluble fiber is found throughout the plant world in foods like legumes, nuts, oats, barley, and certain fruits and veggies like potatoes, corn, carrots, broccoli, apples, and pears.

Insoluble fiber, on the other hand, does not dissolve in water. Instead, it absorbs it, thereby bulking up stool and helping it to move food through the digestive system. When people say that fiber keeps you regular, this is the type they are talking about. It's found in some of the same foods that feature soluble fiber, like potatoes, oats, and broccoli. Other standouts include wheat bran and other whole grains, as well as the skins of certain fruits and veggies.

Not only is fiber linked to a reduced risk of a whole host of chronic ailments—like cardiovascular disease, type 2 diabetes, and colon cancer[26]—it also plays a special role in digestive health. The main way it does this is by feeding our microbiomes. One of the biggest buzzwords in nutrition, *microbiome* refers to the collection of microbes (bacteria, viruses, fungi) that coexist with our bodies—meaning they live in or on them. (Your skin and other organs have microbiomes too, but most of the time, the term refers to the microbiome in your gut.) We often think of microbes as bad things—invaders that wreak havoc and make us sick—but that's true for only some of them. In fact, we have a symbiotic relationship with many microbes, where we act as their host and they aid us in important functions, like helping us digest food, synthesize nutrients, protect against harmful pathogens, and build a robust immune system.[27]

The bacteria living in our large intestines, for example, does the work for us of breaking down soluble fiber. Often referred to as a prebiotic, soluble fiber feeds the gut's good bacteria. Then, as bacteria digests the fiber, the process stimulates the production of beneficial short-chain fatty acids and certain hormones that send signals that we're full.

Low fiber intake, along with a high intake of sugar, fat, and animal protein, is associated with lower levels of diversity in the microbiome when compared to diets rich in minimally processed plant foods. And diversity in your gut is important. While this is an area that's very much evolving in terms of scientific research, studies have suggested connections between our microbiomes and our immune systems, metabolism, mental health, hormones, liver function, and even allergies and obesity.[28, 29, 30] Potentially even our personalities! It's a fascinating area of study, and while too early to draw definitive conclusions on the link between our personalities and our guts, there is evidence to suggest, for example, that highly social people may have more diverse microbiomes.[31, 32, 33]

So how can you get more fiber to feed your microbiome? A diverse, plant-positive diet is the best way because fiber is found only in plants. While people often think of fiber in terms of grains like bran, many fruits, veggies, and legumes are even better sources. Lentils, beans, split peas, green peas, chia seeds, and raspberries are all fiber stars—as are the color stars we recommended in the sidebar.

For optimal health, aim to consume fiber-rich foods every day, ideally at every single meal. Also of note is the fact that a diet heavy in UPFs tends to be low in fiber. As you will recall from the last chapter, that's because when foods are processed, the fiber often gets stripped out. Yet another reason to reach for more real foods when you can!

Gut Helpers Worth Adding

While research suggests that a diet rich in UPFs can suppress diversity in your microbiome, certain foods are known to do the opposite: to feed the good bacteria in your gut and help your microbiome flourish. When looking to add variety—and flavor!—these two categories of gut-helpers are worth seeking out:

Fermented Foods: Fermented foods are one of those food categories that, though processed, are still healthy. In fact, they are among the earliest forms of "processed" foods, used in a variety of cultures around the world for the purpose of extending shelf life and lending flavor to different foods. It turns out that this tried-and-true preservation method has some health benefits as well. The microorganisms that drive fermentation—typically yeast or certain strains of bacteria—act as natural probiotics, adding to the trillions of microorganisms already living in our gut microbiomes and helping them to maintain their diversity and resilience.[34]

Fermented food options include:

- Fermented milk products like yogurt and kefir

- Fermented veggies like kimchi and sauerkraut

- Fermented soy products like miso, tempeh, and natto

- Fermented tea (kombucha)

- (Note: Look for "naturally fermented" products because those are the ones that contain probiotics. In contrast, most pickles you find at the supermarket are pickled using only vinegar and therefore have none.)

Some of these fermented foods may be considered acquired tastes. Natto, for example, is one of the richest sources of vitamin K_2 around and has been linked to a reduced risk of osteoporotic fractures among Japanese women who eat it regularly.[35] But its sticky (some would say slimy) texture and pungent aroma scare some off before they have even tried it. It may be surprising then that its taste is generally mild and slightly nutty. If natto is not for you, give one of the other options a try. There are plenty to choose from. Miso has a mild, salty flavor but without the texture or smell of natto. Kombucha is often paired with other tasty ingredients like ginger or pomegranate. If you allow yourself to experiment, you will almost surely find some fermented foods that you like.

One caution: fermented foods may not be for everyone. They are often not recommended for children under one year old, people with compromised immune systems or histamine intolerance, or those who are pregnant. People with digestive disorders should consult a doctor or dietitian beforehand because, while natural probiotics are recommended for certain conditions, for others they may cause irritation. As always, moderation is key, because fermented foods can upset your stomach if you're not used to them.

If you don't like the taste of fermented foods on their own, cheat a little by trying them in a recipe featuring other foods you enjoy. Our **Twisted Ginger Sesame Dressing** contains miso, and our **Aphrodite Dressing** (page 189) contains yogurt, as do many of our Smoothies with Benefits.

Resistant Starch: Resistant starch, a kind of carbohydrate, provides an awesome array of benefits. It can help you stay regular, maintain a healthy weight and blood sugar levels, lower cholesterol, and reduce the risk of colon cancer—all that *and* it contributes to a healthy gut![36] The latter is due to the fact that it "resists" being digested in the small intestine (hence the name), instead making its way to the large intestine, where it ferments and acts as a prebiotic that feeds beneficial bacteria. Another useful benefit: the fermentation process that breaks down resistant starch happens slowly, so digesting it tends to produce less gas than with other starchy foods. Still, we must warn you that too much can make you gassy and bloated, which is why (as with any changes to your diet) you should start off slowly by consuming small amounts and then work your way up from there.

Options for adding resistant starch include:

- Whole grains like oats, farro, and cooked-and-cooled rice. (Note: Rice that has been cooled is higher in resistant starch and will retain much of that starch when reheated.)
- Legumes, especially lentils and white beans.
- Unripe plantains, green bananas, and green banana flour. (Note: As bananas ripen, the resistant starch turns into regular starch.)

We particularly love green banana flour, which is common in West African, Caribbean, and Central American cooking. It has a mild flavor—not as overly banana-y as you might think—and makes a great addition to any of our smoothie recipes. Start with a teaspoon and see how it sits. Then you can dial up, or dial down, from there depending on how you feel.

Start off your day with a dose of resistant starch by trying our delicious **Savory Farro Bowl** (page 181) or **Banana Oat Mini Muffins** (page 210) for breakfast.

How Much Variety Is in Your Diet?

To help build the habit of adding more plant variety to your meals, we are going to ask you to get counting. We are *not* going to ask you to count the amount you consume of each crucial nutrient we have talked about in this chapter, because that would be next to impossible. Instead, we are going to ask you to simply count your plants.

By counting the number of different plants you eat over the course of a week, you will start to get a picture of how diverse your diet really is. And once you have that picture in mind, you can focus on how to adopt a plant-positive diet by adding a few more here and there to your meals and snacks, not to mention your drinks! (More on that last one in the next chapter.)

We are even going to set a target for you: 30 plants per week. We call this the **30 Plant Challenge**. Why 30? It's not just a random number. In fact, it comes from research done by the American Gut Project, which set out to do the largest microbiome study to date to learn more about how the microbiome affects human health. Among the findings published in 2018 was that "the number of unique plant species that a subject consumes is associated with microbial diversity"[37]—and gut diversity is a good thing, as we talked about earlier. Researchers specifically looked at people who consumed 30 or more plants each week and compared their gut diversity to those who consumed fewer than 10. They found a notable difference.

As we mentioned earlier, research into the microbiome is ongoing, and this study is not the only reason to focus on plant-adding. We mentioned in the Introduction how only 1 in 10 adults (10 percent) are eating enough vegetables, and only a slightly higher percentage (12.3 percent) are eating enough fruits, a fact that puts a tremendous number of people at higher risk of a number of chronic diseases as well as nutrient deficiencies.[38]

FuelUp

We see those percentages as an opportunity because it means there is a lot of room for making a positive impact in how we fuel ourselves and how we feel as a result. It starts with awareness, which is why we are asking you to spend just one week counting your plants to see how much variety you are getting. Then, using the advice in this chapter, you can build from there.

A word of encouragement before you get started, especially if 30 sounds like an impossibly high number: when we enlisted people to test the recipes, strategies, and Blending Lifestyle Plan (Chapter 6) in this book, we had one participant who was certain it would be a struggle to eat so many plants—until she hit 30 on the second day! At first, she thought she would have to eat a bunch of green stuff that she wasn't used to. But it hadn't occurred to her that so many of the things she ate on a regular basis would count: potatoes, bananas, oats (from her morning bowl of oatmeal), peanuts (in her peanut butter), coffee, tea, chocolate. (Yes, chocolate counts—it's from the cacao bean, after all.) That's seven right off the bat. For dinner the first night, she had her staple spaghetti with red sauce (garlic, onion, tomato, basil, oregano—five plants) and upleveled it with a jar of black olives, some capers, and red pepper flakes (three more plants). Just the plants already mentioned added up to 15. She was halfway there, and she had barely made an effort.

The point is that while 30 may sound high, if you pay attention to all the different things you eat, it probably isn't as high as you think. Fruits, vegetables, nuts, seeds, legumes, whole grains, herbs, spices, coffee, and tea all count. So do mushrooms, which are technically fungi, not plants, but they are rich in micronutrients and fiber, so we think they should count. As do the different-colored ingredients we asked you to try earlier in this chapter. Because each color indicates a different nutrient profile, you can count each color separately. That means that if you're at a grocery store or farmer's market and you can find one of those beautiful mixes of white, purple, orange, and green cauliflower florets, that counts as four. White and green asparagus count separately. So do red, orange, yellow, and green bell peppers. So think about how you might paint your plate with as many colors as possible.

And that's not all that counts. A dusting of cinnamon on your morning latte? Count it. A lettuce leaf on your sandwich? Count it.

Parsley and sesame seeds as a garnish on your favorite chicken dish? Count them both. We want you to be generous with yourself *and* generous with your plants!

Plants That Count!

Vegetables	Beans
Fruits	Legumes
Herbs	Whole grains
Spices	Coffee
Nuts	Cacao beans (aka chocolate!)
Seeds	Tea

More *Cheats* to Try to Make Variety the Spice of Your (Dietary) Life

Thirty isn't a magic number. It's simply a useful guidepost to help ensure that you get more of the benefits that plants have to offer, so take it as such. If, on first count, you find you easily make it to 30, then try upleveling in terms of both quantity and quality. Quantity can mean aiming for 35 plants next time, or even 40, or it can mean choosing larger serving sizes. If you counted the one piece of lettuce in your sandwich wrap, then maybe aim for a full serving of lettuce next week. Quality means looking for more nutrient-rich versions of the foods you have chosen. Chocolate counts, as we mentioned, but there are big differences among different chocolate options. Take a look at our breakdown of the different cocoa powder options on page 123, for example, or consider opting for a chocolate bar with less sugar and processed ingredients.

See just how much variety you can manage while still enjoying your food and take note of how these additions make you feel. If, on the other hand, you find you only get to 10, don't beat yourself up about it. Think of that as your starting place and look for opportunities to add. Aim for 15 next week. Or even 12. The real purpose behind counting your plants is to get you thinking differently about the foods you choose and to focus on finding ways to add nutrient-rich fruits, vegetables, nuts, seeds, legumes, and whole grains that work for you.

In fact, much of the benefit of taking the 30 Plant Challenge may be in the act of counting itself. One study found that when people tracked what they ate for eight weeks, they managed to work in two additional servings of veggies *per day* as compared to what they had been eating at the beginning of the study.[39] That's a significant difference. The simple act of paying attention appears to be what made that difference.

As always, let your blender help you. Blending makes it easier to include a greater variety of plants in your everyday meals, because all you have to do is toss them in and hit blend—to make a plant-rich sauce for your meat or fish or a plant-rich dip for a snack, to name just a couple of options. The following tips provide even more ways to add plants.

Think "Little Black Dress" Recipes

"Little black dress," or LBD, recipes are basics that you can accessorize in any number of ways, just like a little black dress that you can change the "flavor" of depending on whether you pair it with heels or high-tops, whether you dress it up with pearls or dress it down with a denim jacket. In much the same way, these recipes can serve as tasty bases for adding a whole range of different plants, depending on what's good, what's available, and what strikes your palate's fancy on a particular occasion. Take pesto, for example. Think about how you might throw half a dozen things into the simplest pesto—basil, pine nuts, garlic, olive oil, Parmesan, and salt—and how easy it could be to add a few more, like parsley, spinach, arugula, mint, tomatoes, walnuts, almonds, kale, artichokes, and/or anything else that sounds good. (We have a whole section of pesto recipes in Chapter 7 that will provide inspiration.)

The same works for hummus. In our recipe chapter, you will find two hummus recipes (**Hooray for Hummus** [page 198] and a colorful **Tri-Color Pepper Hummus** [page 199]), both of which are delicious and nutrient rich on their own. You can take things to the next level by using either as a base for adding plant variety. That's because *soooo* many things taste great on top of or mixed into hummus. Olive tapenade. Roasted chilis, eggplant, and garlic. Caramelized onions. Lemon or lime juice. Toasted pine nuts. Any number of herbs and spices. Even chocolate. (Yes, chocolate hummus is a thing. Don't knock until you try it.) And so much more.

Another classic: chicken soup. A basic version familiar to most of us includes a range of plants: onions, garlic, carrots, celery, dill, parsley (six plants). But there are so many variations, including recipes from practically every corner of the globe. Mexican chicken pozole combines onions, garlic, oregano, cumin, chilis, hominy, and cilantro, and it's often topped with radishes, lime juice, and avocado (10 plants). Filipino *tinola* utilizes onion, ginger, garlic, green papaya, and malunggay leaves (five plants). Italian *brodo di pollo con pastina* adds tomatoes and pasta to classic ingredients. Greek avgolemono includes the addition of lemon juice and rice (as well as egg to make it creamy). Really any kind of soup can serve as an LBD recipe, because it's just so easy to stir in a few more plants like vegetables, herbs, or beans.

This approach works with all kinds of basic smoothie, sauce, dressing, dip, or spreads recipes. It's an easy way to be additive with your plants.

Change Up Your Basics

A lot of us get into habits when it comes to food shopping. We have certain tried-and-true items we buy again and again without thinking much about it. For the sake of diversity, however, it's time to take another look at the staples in your shopping cart and consider trying something new. Maybe you always have peanut butter in your pantry. How about almond butter this time? Or walnut butter? Don't get us wrong: all nut butters are healthy, especially if you choose brands without added sugar and oil. Still, there are differences among the options. Nut butters are relatively comparable in terms of calorie and fat content, but peanut butter has the highest amount of protein. Almond butter, on the other hand, has more fiber and calcium. Walnut butter stands out as a source of omega-3 fatty acids. Mixing things up helps you cover your nutritional bases.

The same thinking can be applied to different plant-based milks, different kinds of lettuce or salad greens, different varieties of potatoes, different chili peppers. Changing things up can also help stave off boredom, helping to ensure you reach for healthy options more often.

Think Mixes

When we say "mixes," we are not talking ultraprocessed mixes like flavored instant-oatmeal packets or cake mixes. We are talking about minimally processed or unprocessed foods that come in a multi-ingredient mix simply because food makers have combined them for your enjoyment and convenience. Think mixed nuts instead of your typical almonds or walnuts; blends of different lettuces and greens (a friend swears by her power-greens mix that includes baby spinach, baby kale, and green and red chard); packages of multicolored carrots or multicolored bell peppers; spice mixes like za'atar (wild thyme, sesame seeds, sumac); or even a basic poultry seasoning (sage, thyme, rosemary, oregano, marjoram, nutmeg, and black pepper). There is so much opportunity for variety in most supermarkets today, so take advantage of the buffet of options on offer. Or, get crafty and make your own mixes. (See our suggested spice mixes on page 133 and our nut and seed blends on pages 129 and 130.)

Recipes to Try Today! A Tasty, Plant-Positive Meal

One of our favorite ways to add plants to our meals is to use Enhanced Broths in our cooking. Broth or stock is used in a wide variety of recipes from soups and stews to casseroles and braised meats. When a recipe calls for something like chicken or beef broth, we like to soup it up (pun intended) by first blending it with veggies and herbs. You can even cook whole grains in Enhanced Broths rather than water. The practice is quick and easy and allows you to not only pack in the nutrients, but also enhance the flavor of your dishes.

This is the kind of base we use for the crowd-pleasing **Mediterranean Chicken Stew** recipe that follows. Remember when we told you that 30 plants per week is easier than you think? Well, this recipe counts for a total of 10 plants if you use both herbs suggested. That means you are already one-third of the way to you goal in just one meal. Serve the stew over rice, and you have just added one more plant!

GOING GREEN BROTH BLEND

Makes about 4 servings

2 zucchinis

2 celery stalks

2 cups spinach or blanched escarole

3 cups chicken, beef, or veggie broth

Add all ingredients to your blender.

Blend until smooth, about 1 minute.

MEDITERRANEAN CHICKEN STEW

Makes about 4 servings

1 cup diced yellow onion

2 cups sliced mushrooms

1 tablespoon extra virgin olive oil

2 boneless, skinless chicken breasts

2 cups Going Green Broth Blend

2 cloves garlic

2 sprigs of rosemary and/or thyme

One 8-ounce can artichoke hearts, rinsed and drained

2 tablespoons capers

1 cup pitted and halved kalamata olives

Brown the onion and mushroom in the olive oil in a good-sized pot.

Add the chicken and brown it on both sides.

Add the broth, garlic, and herbs and cook on medium heat for about 10 minutes.

Give everything a stir and turn the heat down to low. Cover and simmer the stew for an hour.

Give everything another stir. Use a spoon to break up the chicken breast into smaller pieces.

Add the artichokes, capers, and olives. Stir and simmer for another hour.

Check the chicken to make sure it's done to your liking and serve it alone or over brown rice.

Cheat Sheet

3 Ways to Focus on Plant Diversity in Your Diet . . . Right Away!

- **Take the 30 Plant Challenge**
  Count the number of plants you eat over the course of 1 week and see how close you can get to 30 different varieties. Use the worksheet in our Resources section to help you keep track.

- **Focus on Plant-Positivity**
  Whatever number you hit, think about how you can be additive—in terms of not just volume, but also variety: i.e., more, different types of plants more of the time.

- **Paint Your Plate with Color**
  Look for ways to enjoy the full spectrum of color in the plant world for better nutrition *and* enjoyment—after all, it's a gorgeous way to eat!

CHAPTER 4:

Hydration as Fuel

Fuel Up Habit #4

Be more intentional about getting and staying
hydrated, because your life literally depends on it!

When people talk about the habits that lead to good health, they are usually referring to things like eating well, exercising, and getting enough sleep. These are all important, of course, but in our view, there is another that doesn't get enough attention, and that's hydration. We've mentioned macronutrients before, which are the nutrients our bodies need in large quantities to perform basic functions. Traditionally, macros include three broad categories: protein, carbs, and fat. However, some nutrition experts have lately included a fourth: water.

That's because water is required fuel for practically everything our bodies do. We need it to absorb the nutrients in our food. We need it to regulate our body temperature. We need it to power our digestion, detoxification, and elimination processes. We need it to lubricate our muscles and joints. We need it to create homeostasis in the body. We need it for a healthy immune system. Every system in our bodies, practically every function our bodies perform, requires water in one way or another.

And yet, so much of what we consume is actually dehydrating. We've talked about how our diets are high in ultraprocessed foods, which, in addition to the drawbacks we already mentioned, also tend to be dehydrating. Salty foods are dehydrating. Sugary foods are dehydrating. Alcohol, too, is highly dehydrating.

While good hydration is essential for everyone, it's particularly important as we age. A 2020 research paper revealed that most Americans between the ages of 51 and 70, a whopping 65-plus percent of them, are not adequately hydrated. The same study also found that underhydration in this group is a significant risk factor associated with chronic disease, obesity, and even death within three to six years' time.[1] And we are not talking about overt dehydration here, the kind that requires an emergency room visit, but just the kind of mild dehydration that often goes unnoticed.

Even more recently, researchers at the National Institutes of Health published a large study with alarming results: they found a substantial link between poor hydration and early aging.[2] In other words, chronic, low-grade dehydration may accelerate the body's aging process, which increases a person's risk of chronic disease—including heart failure, stroke, lung disease, and dementia. As the leader of the research team, Dr. Natalia Dmitrieva, put it: "Proper hydration may slow down aging and prolong a disease-free life."[3] And who wouldn't want that?

Because Dr. Dana considers this such a crucial topic, she co-authored an entire book on the subject with Gina Bria, head of the Hydration Foundation and an expert on hydration strategies. (If you really want to understand hydration, we suggest you look into that book, called *Quench: Beat Fatigue, Drop Weight, and Heal Your Body through the New Science of Optimum Hydration*.) Through her research for the book and experience working with patients, Dr. Dana has come to the conclusion that being well hydrated may be the **most important thing we can do to prevent and treat chronic disease.**

By the way, everything you have learned up to this point contributes to better hydration, especially that Smoothie with Benefits you are drinking to start off your day. Dr. Dana believes that veggie-packed smoothies are the most hydrating beverage you can consume, even more so than plain water, because they have minerals and fiber that help the water permeate your cells more efficiently. (More on that topic later in this chapter.)

The thing is, people tend to think of hydration as a straightforward topic (just drink a lot of water, right?). Well, it really isn't. So many of us have outdated and ineffective ideas about how to stay hydrated. What's more, so many of us don't realize that what we eat is a big part of it.

Understanding Your Hydration Status

We're going to talk later in this chapter about which hydration strategies work best (hint: your blender can help!) and which are over-rated, but first things first: How do you even know if your body is well hydrated?

Unfortunately, there is some less-than-optimal advice out there. For example, using urine color as a marker is okay[4]—you generally want it to be light yellow or straw colored—but there are reasons why this doesn't always work. It's natural for urine to be darker first thing in the morning, for example. Your urine color may also be affected by things like vitamins (B vitamins, especially), medications, and diet that make this guidance fall somewhat short.

While there is no simple way to measure optimal hydration, the most reliable method Dr. Dana has found is to look at your urine output. You should be urinating every two to three hours while you're awake, but so many of us have purposely trained ourselves not to do this. We spend our days sitting at a desk, or we're frequently on the go, traveling by car or even plane from place to place. We don't want to interrupt what we're doing to go to the bathroom, so we drink less. We need to get out of that habit. It's okay to dial back the liquids once in a while to get through a busy day, but you don't want to make it routine. If you're not urinating every few hours, that's your signal to hydrate more often.

Track Your Hydration Status

Dr. Dana suggests using the tally method to track how many times you urinate throughout the day to gain insight on how hydrated you are.

- Keep a sheet of paper at your desk if that's where you spend most of your time or use a note-taking app on your phone.

- Every time you get up to urinate, mark it down.

- At the end of the day, tally up the number of marks you have made. Remember that you should be urinating every two to three hours while you're awake.

- Do this for a few days and see if you're hitting that mark. And because our hydration status can change with things like the seasons and our activity levels, it's a good idea to do this anytime you feel like you're getting thirsty often.

- If you're not hitting the mark, then make a point of using some of the hydration strategies discussed in this chapter.

Another way to gauge your level of hydration is to **pay attention to your body**. Signals that you might be dehydrated include:

- Headaches
- Constipation
- Brain fog
- Fatigue
- Hunger between meals
- Dry skin
- Stiffness

People often want an exact guideline for how much water to drink each day to avoid these symptoms, but there isn't a formal recommendation recognized by experts, which is why Dr. Dana doesn't like to give one. But she also understands the desire to have something concrete in mind. Later in this chapter, we're going to prompt you to spend a few moments each day checking in with your body and noticing whether you're experiencing any of the symptoms we listed. We do this because so many of us have dehydrating habits and busy lives that are full of stress and distractions. We have grown accustomed to ignoring what our bodies want and need from us. But our bodies are inherently wise, so we need to start listening better.

All that said, sometimes it can help to have a concrete goal in mind while we learn how to listen better. For patients who could really use specific advice, Dr. Dana suggests drinking about 50 percent of their body weight in ounces of water. So, if you weigh 150 pounds, you would drink about 75 fluid ounces spread out over the course of a day (not gulped all at once!). But that's a very general rule. Activity levels, age, genetics, temperature, environment, and medications all have an impact. As does diet. If someone follows a ketogenic or other low-carb diet, for example, Dr. Dana often suggests raising the amount to 75 percent of their weight in ounces. That's because low-carb diets are inherently a diuretic. People who eat this way tend to consume fewer hydrating foods like fruits and vegetables, and less fiber, so they need more water to compensate.

By contrast, Dana once had a patient who needed only a glass or two of water per day. The patient was generally healthy, was not on any dehydrating medications, was only a moderate exerciser (meaning not a ton of sweating), and enjoyed lots of hydrating foods like salads, smoothies, and soups throughout the day. If it was hot outside or she was particularly active one day, she would drink more, but for her, a glass or two of water throughout the day was often enough. The point is that everyone's hydration needs are different, so paying close attention to your body's cues and not overriding them is important. And then, adjusting to suit your body's specific needs is the best advice we can give you.

A Word about Hunger and Hydration

You may have noticed that one of the symptoms of less-than-optimal hydration is hunger between meals. This may sound odd—why would thirst make you hungry?—but once again, it's due to the fact that we're not always great at reading the signals our bodies give us about what they want and need. We need to hone our *interoception*, which is a fancy word to describe our ability to perceive our internal bodily states, like hunger, fullness, and thirst.

A lot of times, what feels like hunger is really our bodies telling us that we're thirsty. Not all the time, but sometimes (and Dr. Dana thinks more often than not). This is likely true if the sensation is paired with a headache or if we suffer from an "afternoon slump." Many people attribute midafternoon energy drains to low blood sugar and reach for a snack. That may be what's happening, but it's perhaps just as likely that they could simply use a glass of water.

Dr. Dana likes to tell people that, when they feel hungry in between meals—or if they feel any of the other symptoms on the list, like grogginess or headaches—to **start with water**: drink a glass of water and see what happens. If you still feel hungry, then have a snack—ideally a hydrating snack like one of our Salad Shooters—but it's always good practice to try water first. Dr. Dana has found that many people are surprised by how often this simple fix works.

It's our belief that no matter your size, no matter what chronic conditions you live with, fueling yourself in the way we are recommending in this book can have a positive impact—on how you feel, on how much energy you have, on your health and well-being overall. This is particularly true when it comes to being well hydrated. Recent research also suggests that water may be an effective way to both prevent and treat obesity and metabolic syndrome,[5] a collection of conditions that includes high blood pressure, high blood sugar, and high triglyceride counts, which puts people at higher risk of heart disease, stroke, and diabetes. A 2020 study done on mice found that water suppressed the antidiuretic hormone vasopressin, which has been linked to obesity and metabolic syndrome. Research in this area is ongoing, but experts are currently looking at whether a simple increase in water intake can make a real difference. Dr. Dana believes it can, and, as the saying goes, it certainly couldn't hurt!

This is not a diet book, as we have tried to make clear, but if you are trying to lose weight for health reasons, it may be worth focusing more closely on your hydration status. The same may be true if you have a "sweet tooth" or a "salt tooth" and are looking to cut back. More research is needed to determine if the kind of "water therapy" that worked for mice can also work for humans, but we have found anecdotally that being well hydrated can be an effective tool for curbing cravings. When Colin goes out to dinner or to a party where he knows there will be alcohol and less healthy fare, he likes to make use of the pregaming strategy we talked about earlier by drinking a small, greens-filled smoothie an hour or two before he leaves. That way he shows up feeling both hydrated and nourished. He still indulges, but the practice helps him consume a little less. It's something he's done for years because it works so well for him.

Try our **Popeye's Passion Salad Shooter** (page 202) or **Parsley Perfect Salad Shooter** (page 203) to load up on nourishment and hydration before going out on the town.

Food Can Hydrate

Once you have a sense of your hydration levels, the natural next question is: What works to stay hydrated? There's some sketchy information out there about this topic as well. For example, you have surely heard the advice to drink eight glasses of water a day. This is a myth that will not die. It's unclear why the advice has become so ubiquitous or where it even started, though some believe it began with the U.S. Food and Nutrition Board's statement way back in 1945 saying that people need about 2.5 liters of water a day. That's the equivalent of about 84.5 ounces, so eight standard drinking glasses (typically 10 to 16 ounces) would cover it. Of course, even in 1945, the advice didn't make sense, because the very next sentence in the board's statement was that most of that amount would come from food.[6] Yes, many of the foods we eat count toward our hydration.

Perhaps the advice stuck because it's easy to picture, if not exactly easy to follow. (Have you ever tried drinking eight full glasses of water in a day? It's a lot.) Instead of counting glasses, a better way to stay hydrated is to do what we talked about in the last chapter: count your plants! Foods can be either hydrating or dehydrating, but the one reliably hydrating category of foods is plants. Think back to all the different kinds of plants we asked you to start adding to your meals—fruits, vegetables, nuts, legumes, seeds. They all provide hydration. In fact, plants can be anywhere from 80 to 98 percent water.

Many people are dismissive of iceberg lettuce, for example, saying that darker green lettuces are far better for you. While it's true that darker lettuces like romaine and watercress contain more micronutrients, phytonutrients, and fiber, it's not like iceberg contains none of these things. What's more, the reason iceberg has fewer nutrients is because it has a higher water content instead. Iceberg lettuce is about 96 percent water! That's what makes it so crisp and crunchy. We hope that you will enjoy a wide *variety* of greens, from pale to dark on the color spectrum, but don't let anyone tell you that iceberg can't count as one of them. It's highly hydrating, low in calories, and has a bit of nutrition all at the same time. Dr. Dana finds that people love it when she tells them this fact!

It's not just the fact that plants contain water that makes them so hydrating. It's also the nature of the water inside them. We've said this before, but we'll say it again: nature has our backs. When we get our water from plants, it comes with added benefits that make it even more hydrating than water alone. Fiber is a good example. In the last chapter, we talked about how this chronically underconsumed nutrient has all sorts of advantages, from feeding the good bacteria in our microbiomes to slowing down digestion so we feel full longer. It also aids hydration because the soluble fiber in plants attracts and absorbs water. When we digest that fiber, the water is then released into our cells more slowly. Have you ever drunk a glass of water and felt like it went right through you? That's less likely to happen when you get your water from plants, because the fiber helps it stay in our bodies longer.

Soluble Fiber: A Hydration Star

Soluble fiber is *hydrophilic*, or water-loving, in nature (as opposed to insoluble fiber, which doesn't absorb water). Because seeds like chia seeds and flax are fiber dense with soluble fiber, they can expand to hold a high proportion of water. That's why when you add liquid to dry-looking chia or flax seeds, they soak it up and turn into a sticky, gelatinous pudding! You can take advantage of the hydrophilic quality of soluble fiber by adding seeds to your water. Start by mixing a teaspoon into herbal tea or water and then consider increasing the amount if you tolerate them well. (Remember, large amounts of fiber can be hard on the stomach if you're not used to it!) Or, try these seeds in one of our recipes. Several of our smoothies, our Salad Shooters, and even our Matcha Pudding dessert (page 205) include hydrating seeds among their ingredients.

Another way that nature has our backs is by combining minerals, including electrolytes, together with water in the plants we eat. In basic terms, electrolytes are minerals that conduct electrical energy when dissolved in water. Each of our cells is like a tiny battery that carries an electrical charge, so we need electrolytes for proper cell function. It feels like electrolyte water has been all the rage in recent years, but what gets lost in the marketing is that you don't need a powder or a special (read: more costly) bottled water to get your electrolytes. Common electrolytes include potassium, calcium, magnesium, and sodium, all of which can be found in varying amounts in different plants.

Once again, you are already enjoying the hydrating benefits of plants if you have been having your smoothie a day and eating more plants like we suggested in earlier chapters. You're also helping your hydration status if you have been swapping out some UPFs for more natural, whole foods. So, this is just more reason to continue those habits we have been talking about all along. Beyond that, we're going to offer you a few more ways to be more intentional about hydration.

Case Study: Jeremy

As a physician's assistant, Jeremy already understood the importance of drinking water and routinely talked with his patients about the difference it can make to their health and well-being. And he practiced what he preached, carrying with him a water bottle that he would drink from and refill multiple times a day. It hadn't occurred to him that there could be more effective ways to hydrate than simply drinking water until he read *Quench*, the book Dr. Dana co-authored about the science of optimum hydration. After that, he decided to give some of the advice a try.

The changes he made were really quite small and easy to do. Instead of drinking plain water, he added chia seeds, sea salt, and fresh lemon or lime juice to his water bottle and drank two of those a day, as well as a third bottleful of plain water. Jeremy was already healthy and fit when he decided to do this, so you might think there was little room for improvement in how he felt. In fact, he described being "shocked" by the results!

Jeremy practices calisthenics five days a week and had been doing it long enough that he had a clear sense of how long he could typically hold different positions. But, after just a few days of hydrating differently, he was able to blow past those benchmarks.

"On my *last* set, when I am the most tired and my time is the shortest before my form falters, I had a significant increase in endurance," he explained. He was able to hold a wall handstand 165 percent longer than before (yes, he did the math), and another position called the back lever—which already requires a significant amount of back and core strength—700 percent longer.

"I went through every conceivable variable that could in any way play into this and eliminated them all," he told Dr. Dana in disbelief. "The *only* variable that changed was the hydration program. Wow!"

Even Dr. Dana found the results encouraging, and she was already well convinced of the benefits of becoming better hydrated. After all, if it can have that kind of effect on an already-fit person's exercise regimen, think of the potential it can have for the rest of us—on our energy levels, our stamina, and our ability to fuel ourselves through our busy days!

Infuse Your Water

Eating more plants is an effective way to stay hydrated, but that doesn't mean you shouldn't drink *any* water. You probably won't need eight full glasses to meet your hydration needs, but you are going to require some liquids throughout the day.

Dr. Dana has been stressing the importance of hydration for years now, and one of the problems she has found is that a lot of people simply don't like to drink water. They don't enjoy the taste (or more aptly, the tastelessness), and they think of it as a chore—something they should do but don't really want to do and therefore aren't motivated to do until they get really thirsty. The problem is that **if you wait until you're thirsty to drink, you are already dehydrated.**[7] Thirst is the definition of dehydration!

This is one of the reasons why Colin created a hydration system to go with his Beast blender, one that allows people to infuse their water with flavor. By pulsing ingredients like mint, ginger, lemon, strawberries, or whatever else you enjoy, and then letting those ingredients infuse your water (in the same way you might infuse water with tea leaves), you get a number of added benefits that you don't get from plain water. First, it gives you an extra hit of nutrition—vitamins, minerals, electrolytes, phytonutrients, and fiber—from the plants you add. Second, it makes your water taste good—and that may be the most important reason of all.

One of the main principles of habit-building is that you are more likely to do something if you enjoy doing it. This doesn't work with everything. Kids still need to get in the habit of brushing their teeth even though they may hate doing it. But, for many people, focusing on enjoyment can work quite well when it comes to getting into a hydration habit. Because let's face it: people love flavored water. It has become a huge and growing market over the past decade, with companies offering a wide range of flavors for both still and sparkling options from straightforward lemon or lime to the exotic, like lychee, cactus rose, or strawberry hibiscus.

This tip works for Colin, who doesn't really like the taste of plain water and finds that a little flavoring makes it much easier to drink. It has also worked for Dr. Dana's husband, Henry, who was a regular Diet Coke and Fresca drinker when they met. She doesn't mind if a generally healthy person has a soda once in a while, but she didn't love that he was drinking ultraprocessed beverages laden with artificial sweeteners practically all day, every day. He would often grab a two-liter bottle of soda in the morning and drink it throughout the afternoon. It was his main liquid. One day she got him to try Spindrift, a brand of sparkling water with a squeeze of real fruit juice. They have a grapefruit flavor that was reminiscent of Fresca, and Henry liked it so much, he was willing to swap it for his usual soda. It turned out that soda wasn't such a hard habit to break when he had something he liked just as well to replace it. He still has a soda once in a while, but only when he's out. He no longer feels the need to keep it in the fridge at home. Breaking ingrained habits isn't always so easy, of course, but when it can be, why not take advantage of it?

Even better than buying flavored water in our opinion—yummier, cheaper, and better for the environment because it means fewer plastic bottles or aluminum cans—is to use your blender to make your own Enhanced Water Infusions to suit your tastes. It's naturally flavored water, instead of water with artificial flavors or sweeteners, and it also uplevels the nutrients in your drink.

Enhanced Water Infusions are a simple cheat for keeping yourself fully fueled throughout the day, one that can make your hydration habit that much more interesting, tasty, and fun. We have an entire section of recipes for enhancing your water in Chapter 7. You can even infuse frozen water, otherwise known as popsicles, in the summer. (For frozen water infusions that are not only hydrating but also feel like a treat, try our **Blackberry Freezer Pops** or use up leftover fruit in our **Refrigerator Cleanup Fruit Pops** on page 208.)

And don't let the enjoyment stop there. Get a fancy water bottle or special water glass that will make you smile when you use it. Buy a fun, reusable straw, as most people prefer to sip their drinks. Do whatever works to make hydrating more appealing, and you will be more likely to keep up the habit.

Try an Enhanced Water Infusion

To support the habit of being more intentional about hydration, try making your own flavored water to enjoy throughout the day. We have a selection of recipes to choose from in Chapter 7, but what follows is a favorite to get you started. It pairs blueberries—which have the reputation of being among the healthiest fruits thanks to their high antioxidant content—with basil, also known as the "royal herb," which also offers a healthy dose of micro- and phytonutrients. This classic flavor combination is sure to please practically any palate!

BASIL BLUEBERRY DELIGHT ENHANCED WATER INFUSION

1 small handful of blueberries
2 basil leaves

Pulse the ingredients in your blender until they are combined but still chunky.

Spoon pulsed ingredients into an infuser, tea ball, or fillable tea bag and submerge in water. You can also simply spoon the mixture into a glass and pour water over the top if you don't mind some chewable bits in your drink!

Enjoy!

Plan Your Hydration

The best way to ensure that you are hydrating fully is to plan for it before you need it. Because, don't forget: if you wait until you're thirsty to hydrate, you are already dehydrated.

To make it easy, we have created a schedule for you. Everyone's day is different, so we have made the schedule flexible enough to adapt to your circumstances, whether you're a typical nine-to-fiver, you work nights, your schedule varies from week to week, or whatever else might apply. We suggest you **build three hydration breaks into your day** to help you become more intentional about hydrating. During those breaks—short ones, we promise!—you will focus not just on drinking liquids, but also on checking in with your body. And maybe taking the opportunity to add in a little movement. This isn't an exercise book, of course, but we all know that exercise is important for good health. What not everyone realizes, however, is that even simple movements can have real benefits. A recent study found that just 22 minutes of activity a day can compensate for the harms caused by sitting for extended periods, as so many of us do, and you can break that up into five-minute increments four or five times a day.[8] So, as long as you are taking a break already, consider moving a little bit, stretching, twisting, and walking around the room even if you can't get outside. You will find that it actually makes you more productive.

Your Daily Hydration Break Schedule

- When you wake up: Start your day with water.

- Midway between breakfast and lunch:
  Take a hydration break.

- Midway between lunch and dinner:
  Take a hydration break.

To help you establish this habit, we suggest that you set a daily timer on your phone or computer to alert you when it's time to hydrate. You may also want to plan ahead and have your water ready, especially if you opt for an Enhanced Water Infusion. And if you want flavored water but don't have time to make an infusion, then simply cut up some fruit and pop it in a glass. The point is to make these breaks as easy and enjoyable as possible.

When You Wake Up: Start Your Day with Water

First thing, before you do anything else, drink 1 large glass of water.

Colin likes to drink electrolyte water (see our recipe at the end of this chapter) because he works out in the mornings, but you can choose lemon water or another flavor infusion, water with a pinch of salt for electrolytes, or just plain water. It really doesn't matter, in our opinion. We are aware that a lot of people swear by lemon water, for instance, even though the benefits are sometimes overstated. Still, lemon juice will provide an added hit of important micronutrients like vitamin C, so if you like it, then go for it. If it feels like too much trouble to cut up some fruit while you're still groggy, then forget it. If water feels too boring, mix things up by adding ginger, strawberries, cucumber, or whatever strikes your fancy. Go with whatever is going to work best for you in the mornings.

Do this *before coffee*—not because we're anti caffeine, but to help ensure you begin your day well hydrated. When you sleep, your body does most of its detoxing. That's why your first urination of the day tends to be darker in color—it has a higher concentration of waste products. Starting your day with water helps flush out your system and replace the water you used up while sleeping.

Myths about Hydration

There are two stubborn myths about hydration out there. We have already talked about the first one, which is that you need to drink eight glasses of water a day. The other is that coffee dehydrates you. This one is only mostly false. Coffee can be dehydrating if you have a lot of it, but you can drink up to 4 cups of coffee a day with no diuretic effect,[9] meaning the liquid still counts as hydration. This is true of caffeinated beverages in general, but it doesn't mean we recommend you drink them all day long or that they should be your only choice of beverage. While daily caffeine intake of up to 300 milligrams is not dehydrating (the amount per serving varies by beverage, but that equals roughly 9 cans of Coke or 4 cups of coffee), it can still cause jitters and indigestion and have a negative impact on things like sleep, blood pressure, and anxiety. While we both drink coffee in the morning, infused water is still our preferred beverage for drinking throughout the day.

Midway between Breakfast and Lunch: Take a Hydration Break

Drink 1 glass of enhanced water.

For many of us who are nine-to-fivers, this will be around 10 A.M., but you can adjust the time according to your own natural waking and eating timeline. Also, consider what might get in the way—maybe that's when you meet with your team at work, or you're usually in the car on the way to pick up your kid from nursery school. Plan around those potential barriers before setting your alarm so it's that much easier to stick to the habit.

For this hydration break, you can opt for one of our Enhanced Water Infusions or herbal tea, either hot or cold. In a pinch, a simple glass of water will do, with or without cut-up fruit. We have been encouraging you all along to pay attention to your body, so this is a good time to check in to see how you feel:

- Feeling stiff? Try a few movements or take a short walk. Even if you're not feeling stiff, this can be a good time to work in some neck rolls, twists, and stretches to wake up your body and your brain.

- Feeling snackish or low on energy? Try water first. If you're still hungry after that, have one of our satiating snack options. (See page 198 for suggestions.)

Midway between Lunch and Dinner: Take a Hydration Break

Drink 1 glass of enhanced water.

At around 3 o'clock in the afternoon (or whatever time works for your schedule), follow the same advice above: Take a few moments to gauge what your body wants and needs from you, move around a little, and focus on hydration.

More Cheats to Try

If you have done everything that we have talked about so far and you still feel like you could use some extra hydration, try the following tips:

Drink a Glass of Water before Meals

If you have trouble remembering to hydrate, pairing the practice with something you already do regularly can be an effective strategy. You know you're going to stop throughout the day to eat, so take the opportunity to also focus on hydration. By drinking the water *before* you eat, it can also help ensure that you are not confusing your thirst cues with your hunger ones.

Consider Adding Electrolytes

Dana has had numerous patients complain that, even though they drink water all day long, they're still thirsty! If you find yourself thirsty again soon after drinking water, try adding electrolytes. This can be in the form of one of our electrolyte refresher recipes, a store-bought electrolyte powder, or even a pinch of sea salt. You may also want to try this when you sweat more than usual, like during intense workouts or on hot days, both of which cause you to lose water and electrolytes more quickly.

Even just adding a pinch of salt can help because both sodium and chloride, the elements that make up salt, are electrolytes, which play a key role in drawing water into your cells. It's a way to help your body absorb water more efficiently, thereby preventing dehydration. Dana has seen this simple solution help alleviate muscle cramps and restore energy in a number of patients.

Some may hear this advice and worry about the added sodium. After all, it has been drilled into us that too much salt is generally bad for us and can raise our blood pressure. The truth is that otherwise healthy people probably don't need to be overly worried about added salt, especially not the pinch we are suggesting here. And while doctors have long recommended low-salt diets for patients with high blood pressure, heart failure, or other cardiac issues, even the research behind that advice is not definitive.[10] Some research even suggests that too little sodium can worsen heart disease in some people.[11] If you are worried or have heart issues, the best advice is to consult your doctor.

The Skinny on Salt

You may have noticed that there are a wide range of salt options for sale these days, and it's important to note that they are not the same. Your typical table salt has been processed to remove minerals that bond with salts in nature, and it also includes additives like anticaking or conditioning agents. That's why we recommend natural **sea salt or rock salt** instead. These options are less processed and contain beneficial trace minerals like potassium, magnesium, and calcium. A brand we like is Redmond Real Salt, an unrefined sea salt that boasts more than 60 different naturally occurring trace minerals.

There Is Such a Thing as Too Much Water

One last caution: don't overdo the plain water. Too much can upset your electrolyte balance, causing you to lose necessary minerals, especially sodium. The condition is called *hyponatremia* or "water intoxication," and it crops up in the headlines every so often, like with the ill-conceived Water Gallon Challenge that went viral. But it's no joke. Water intoxication is a serious condition that can cause fainting, seizures, and even be fatal in rare cases. In 2023, actress Brooke Shields suffered a grand mal seizure after overhydrating and had to be rushed to the hospital.

Electrolyte levels in the body are constantly in flux based on what we consume and how much we sweat, but most of the time, our kidneys are remarkably good at making adjustments to keep us balanced. Those levels can get out of whack, however, when we quickly drink too much plain water and sweat excessively at the same time. We lose electrolytes through sweat, so combining that with an excess of water can overwhelm the kidneys. It's not common, but it does happen, especially to athletes like marathon runners and those training in hot weather. Dr. Dana has also seen it among hot-yoga practitioners and even those who are trying to be healthy by carrying around a water bottle and sipping excessive amounts of plain water throughout the day.

Recipe to Try Today!
Make Your Own Electrolyte Water

No need for pricey bottled versions or processed powders when you make your own tasty electrolyte water at home. Salt is made up of sodium and chloride, which are both electrolytes, and citrus juice contains small amounts of others, like calcium, potassium, and magnesium. A sweetener is also included for more than just flavor. While complex carbs high in fiber are generally the healthiest choice, quick-digesting carbs, like the honey or maple syrup used here, are better for fueling workouts.

LEMON LIME ELECTROLYTE REFRESHER

Makes about 2 servings

2 cups cold water
1 lemon wedge, pith and peel included
1 lime wedge, pith and peel included
2 pinches salt
2 tablespoons honey or maple syrup

Cheat Sheet

3 Ways to Be More Intentional about Hydration . . . Right Away!

- **Pay Attention to Your Hydration Status**
  Use Dr. Dana's tally system to find out if you are urinating every 2 to 3 hours while you are awake. Notice symptoms you may be having related to hydration, like headaches, stiffness, and feeling hungry in between meals, and, before reaching for a snack or a pain reliever, try drinking a glass of water to see if symptoms alleviate.

- **Use Food as Hydration**
  If you are following the cheats from previous chapters, you are already doing this! A smoothie a day is hydrating. Adding plants to your meals is hydrating. Here is one more reason to keep it up and perhaps add a few more plants throughout the week.

- **Add Hydration Breaks to Your Day**
  Build 3 short breaks into your day, times when you check in with your body and enjoy a glass of water or an infusion. These breaks don't have to be long. Even just a minute or two will do the trick!

  ✓ When You Wake Up
  ✓ Midway between Breakfast and Lunch
  ✓ Midway between Lunch and Dinner

CHAPTER 5:

Play with Your Food

Fuel Up Habit #5

Make healthy eating more sustainable
by getting creative with your food.

So far in this book, we have walked you through several Fuel Up Habits that will keep you feeling nourished and fully fueled to lead the life you want. But we're not blind to the fact that these habits may be different from what you're used to and that change of this kind—of any kind, really—can be challenging. This is true even when you understand why the change is important and how, with the help of your blender, you can make it easier and less time-consuming to adopt.

With that in mind, we would like to suggest a way to address any challenges you encounter in adopting or sustaining these habits. We would like to suggest that you approach this new way of eating with a spirit of creativity, flexibility, and *play*. We want you spend more time playing with your food as a way of opening yourself up to trying new things, because it has the potential to enhance both your food choices and your happiness.

That last part may sound like a stretch, but there is research showing that a healthy amount of openness to new experiences, what's called *neophilia*, is associated with happiness.[1] And food can serve as a kind of low-hanging fruit in this way (pun intended!). It is an accessible area of our lives in which we can feel free to play, experiment, and try new things.

If you're thinking, *I like what I like and nothing's gonna change that*, consider how your taste buds have already changed over the course of your life. When you were a kid, there were probably all sorts of foods that seemed too gross or too intolerable to even try. Because of the taste, smell, look, or some combination of all three, kids commonly reject things like fish, wine, beer, and fragrant cruciferous vegetables like broccoli, Brussels sprouts, and cauliflower. Coffee is another example of something that tastes bitter and awful to many people the first time they try it, which is why they start out drinking it with cream and sugar rather than black. Dr. Dana drank her coffee with Sweet'N Low for years, until one week she decided to experiment with fasting and the plan she was on allowed only black coffee. She was apprehensive at first, but found the switch was easier than expected. After the fast, she found her tastes had changed. She never went back to the Sweet'N Low.

The truth is that our taste buds evolve throughout our lifetimes whether we want them to or not. Our senses of taste and smell typically become more dulled as we age, so what we like may continue to shift in spite of ourselves.[2] But as we discussed earlier, we can also help create change for our own benefit. Our graduating Smoothie with Benefits levels are based on this principle. By starting with ones that are more fruit-forward and then progressively adding more vegetables as you go, they are designed to help your tastes evolve.

On your current journey of cheating your way to good health, playing with your food and being open to trying new things will be useful in several ways. They can help you to:

- **Find solutions to food reactions you might encounter** by experimenting to better understand what's happening in your body and how the issue can be addressed.

- **Examine your relationship with food** and hopefully form a more beneficial one.

- **Enjoy your food more,** which is the best healthy eating cheat of them all!

Finding Solutions to Food Reactions

When adopting new healthy eating habits or introducing new foods, people sometimes find they don't feel quite as well as they expected. One couple who tried the 7-Day Beast Blending Lifestyle Plan you will find in the next chapter discovered they had very different reactions to starting their days with a Smoothie with Benefits. The husband felt energized and loved that breakfast came together more quickly than his typical bowl of oatmeal. The wife, however, enjoyed the blends but found she had some mild gastrointestinal issues like acid reflux. A bit of experimenting led her to discover that the portion size was just a bit too large. She found that a two-thirds portion worked better for her.

**Some issues that might come up for you
over the course of this book could be:**

I get hungry again soon after my morning blend.

I experience uncomfortable gas and/or bloating.

I experience acid reflux.

I experience stomach upset or constipation.

I get tired after drinking my blend.

I experience headaches.

There can be a variety of reasons for each of these issues, including simply too much change too quickly. However, symptoms like these don't necessarily mean you should abandon course and go back to how you were eating before. A better approach is to be mindful of how you feel and use it as an opportunity to find out more about how your body works. Being open, curious, and willing to try different remedies can be helpful here.

If you experience one or more of the issues listed above, consider some of the likely culprits that follow, along with our suggestions for what you can do to feel better:

Issues with Portion Size

May cause: Hunger, headaches, or fatigue after eating, if portions are too small. On the other hand, feeling too full, weight gain, and/or experiencing GI issues like bloating and acid reflux, if portions are too large.

When you're not used to having your breakfast in a glass, it's not always easy to tell if you're packing too much or too little into your meal. Our Smoothie with Benefits recipes are portioned for an average eater, but most people aren't strictly average. People in smaller bodies tend to require fewer calories and therefore smaller meals. Highly active people tend to require more calories to fuel themselves and therefore larger meals. Some people wake up hungry, while others prefer smaller breakfasts. You will want to take note of how you feel after trying our recipes and adjust to what works best for your body.

What to do: If you find you crave a snack soon after breakfast and that's unusual for you, or if you end up tired or headachy, try increasing the protein in your morning blend by 10 percent and see how you feel. If you're a highly active person, especially in the morning, you might even try a slightly bigger portion overall.

On the other hand, if you end up having any of the GI symptoms described, try cutting back to a three-quarters portion and see if the symptoms alleviate and you still feel satisfied. Another option to try is to have your smoothie meal for lunch. For some people, a fiber- and protein-filled meal doesn't sit as well first thing in the morning, but they might digest it just fine a few hours later.

Excess Fiber

May cause: Bloating, gas, stomach pain, diarrhea, or constipation.

The Fuel Up way of eating is full of plants and therefore full of fiber. As we have already discussed, fiber is good for you for so many reasons, and most of us aren't getting enough of it. But fiber can also be a bit tricky. It's often an effective remedy for constipation, but for some people, it makes it worse.[3] If you do encounter problems consuming more fiber, just know that it's too important to simply delete from your diet without trying to find a way to make things better.

What to do: Often issues with fiber stem from the fact that you have added too much too quickly, and your body is having trouble adjusting. Cut back and see how you feel. When you start to feel better, begin dialing up the amount gradually. You might also find that your body accommodates fiber better when it comes in the form of cooked veggies rather than raw. Another tip is to make sure you drink plenty of water, which helps with the digestive process. Don't ignore persistent symptoms, however, as they can be a sign of serious GI issues like small intestinal bacterial overgrowth (SIBO) or Crohn's disease. If symptoms don't subside, see a doctor.

Food Allergies

May cause: Itching; hives; swelling of lips, face, or throat; wheezing and trouble breathing; anaphylactic shock.

First, let's talk about how food allergies are different from food intolerances, because either can cause problems, but they are two very different things. Allergies are an immune system response, where the body views the allergen as an uninvited guest to the party who needs to be dealt with immediately. Symptoms tend to come on quickly and can sometimes be life-threatening.

In Dr. Dana's experience, it's rare to find a food allergy in an adult, but it happens every once in a while, and it can make a real difference to someone's health when treated. If you're trying new foods that you have never tried before, it's possible that you might come across an undiagnosed allergy.

Common allergens include nuts, eggs, shellfish, and soy.

What to do: Suspected allergies merit a trip to the doctor for testing. Many allergens can be diagnosed through blood tests, and if an allergy is discovered, the offending food should be avoided.

Food Intolerances

May cause: GI symptoms like gas, bloating, diarrhea, or constipation; skin reactions like acne, psoriasis, or eczema; issues with mental clarity including fatigue, brain fog, and migraines; respiratory issues like nasal congestion; joint issues, including pain and stiffness. Food intolerance symptoms can be so diverse that Dr. Dana likes to say, "You name it, and it could potentially be the result of a food intolerance."

Unlike allergies, food intolerances—which happen when foods aren't broken down properly in the body—are not life-threatening, but their symptoms can have a real impact on you over time. Food intolerances affect an estimated 20 percent of the population,[4] but because they can manifest in different ways and the symptoms aren't typically as dire as they are with allergies, they often go undiagnosed and untreated.

The most common sensitivities that Dr. Dana comes across are gluten, dairy, soy, eggs, and corn.

What to do: Try a simple elimination diet. This is not the kind of diet that has you counting calories and aiming to drop pounds, but rather a structured eating plan that involves temporarily removing specific foods or food groups suspected of causing intolerance symptoms. By systematically reintroducing those foods, one at a time, and monitoring your body's reactions, you can pinpoint which ones trigger your symptoms. (See the Resource section for more information on how to do this.)

Drop in Blood Sugar

May cause: Fatigue, headaches, energy crashing after eating, dizziness, brain fog.

Something called "reactive hypoglycemia" can occur for people who are nondiabetic after eating a meal high in carbs. The symptoms that occur are a result of a drop in blood sugar. If you are adding a lot of fruit to your morning Smoothie with Benefits and find yourself having these kinds of symptoms within four hours afterward, reactive hypoglycemia may be what's happening.

What to do: Try dialing back the amount of fruit in your smoothie, maybe adding additional protein like nuts or seeds and/or a healthy fat like avocado in its place. You can also try choosing lower-glycemic fruits like berries, peaches, green apple, kiwi, and cantaloupe. As with all reactions surrounding food, if symptoms persist, consult your doctor, because reactive hypoglycemia can signal an underlying health condition and may be a risk factor for diabetes later in life.

General Tips for Troubleshooting Food Issues

- **Introduce new foods gradually.** If you're not used to eating greens, for example, start with a small handful in your morning blend and work your way up. If fiber hasn't been a big part of your diet, you're going to want to start with a small amount and build from there. Otherwise, you risk gastrointestinal symptoms like cramps and bloating.

- **Substitute as needed.** One of the many benefits of blending is that it's easy to sub things in or out depending on what works for your body and your taste buds, as well as what's available to you. If you're on a diet for health reasons, like a low-FODMAP or a diabetic-friendly, low-sugar plan, blending recipes are easily adaptable to meet specific requirements. The same is true if you really don't like something in a recipe or can't find it at the store. Refer back to Chapter 1 for some examples of common substitutions you might want to make.

- **Listen to your body.** If you feel any sort of symptom, do not simply ignore it or take a pill to alleviate it. Instead, take a moment to consider what might be going on. A food journal can be a useful tool here if symptoms are recurring. It can help you identify patterns and experiment with different options to see if some things make you feel better or worse than others. Our bodies have real wisdom to share with us about what they need and want to function at their best, but they can only share that wisdom with us if we take time to listen.

Building a Better Relationship with Food

Playing with your food and trying new things requires a spirit of openness and curiosity, which has another advantage: it can help us examine our relationship with food and better understand the choices we make around it.

What we choose to eat or not eat isn't just about providing fuel for our bodies. People eat for all sorts of reasons. Out of habit. Out of boredom. For comfort—comfort food is a whole category of foods for a reason. As celebration—it's hard to think of birthdays without thinking about birthday cake. As ritual or tradition—many holidays and religious rituals have foods attached to them, or the absence of food in the form of fasts. As a reaction to emotions like fear, anxiety, stress, even excitement or happiness.

In the same way that we have seen an array of physical reactions when we ask people to eat differently, we have also seen a variety of psychological reactions. Again, it's worth taking some time to investigate those reactions and consider what you can do to remove, minimize, or even accommodate the barriers that can make it more difficult to cheat your way to good health.

Some reactions we have encountered include:

I don't have time for this.
I don't want to give up my favorites.
I don't like vegetables.
I don't like "health food."
This way of eating will leave me hungry.
I just want to do things my own way.

If you find yourself coming up with objections like these, especially if they arise before you have even tried our way of eating, here are some tactics that can help.

Ask Yourself Some Questions

Say you just had breakfast, and an hour later you find yourself getting up to find a snack. Have you ever stopped to ask yourself why you want that snack? What, exactly, are you feeding?

Most of us engage in a behavior like this on instinct, without thinking much about it, but when we talked to people who were following our Beast Blending Lifestyle Plan, we received an interesting range of answers about why they reach for a snack.

- One person found that he was simply hungry by midmorning. For him, increasing his portion by just a little, as well as the amount of protein in his smoothie, made a difference.

- One woman noticed that she did this only on weekdays, not weekends, which made her realize that her morning snack was more about taking a break and relieving some of the stress of her job than it was about hunger. She decided to get up from her desk and try a few stretches instead.

- Another man decided he snacked for the social experience. He and some of his colleagues had a habit of meeting midmorning to chat while munching on whatever snacks or breakfast meeting items had been left in the breakroom. He enjoyed it, so he kept doing it, but he did become more conscious of what he chose to eat. He even got a group together to approach the HR department about providing healthier options, because it was something they all wanted available to them.

- A mother of a new baby found that she often reached for a snack after putting her son down for a nap, mostly as a source of comfort or sometimes even a reward if it had been a hard night without a lot of sleep. Understanding that led her to make different choices at times. Sometimes she still had a snack, but at other times, she found more comfort in taking a few moments for herself by flipping through a magazine or texting with a friend.

Asking yourself questions like, **How am I feeling right now? What am I looking to satisfy? or even, How will this nourish me?** can be enlightening. The point is not to judge what you do or beat yourself up about it. The point is to invoke a bit of curiosity about what's behind the choices you make, and then, perhaps, to wonder whether those choices are having the desired effect. For example, if relief from anxiety or stress is what you need, then is a snack the best way to achieve it? Is there something that might work better?

You don't have to ask these questions every time you eat, and the answers don't even have to lead to changes in behaviors. But our choices around food can be a telling reflection of how we are feeling, what we are thinking, what habits we have gotten into, what we value, and even what our biases are. Having a better understanding of our food choices can only lead to a better understanding of ourselves.

Case Study: Devin

Devin, who is in his 30s and works in film and television production, decided he wanted to make some changes to the way he was eating, because it felt like his body was telling him that he needed to. He regularly felt headachy, bloated, and sluggish. He was often so tired that he would fall asleep at 3 o'clock in the afternoon. He had been relying on energy drinks to give him a boost, but he didn't like the way they made him feel. He felt anxious much of the time, and he attributed it to those drinks.

"My body, I just feel, wasn't producing the energy that I needed," he explained. He also realized that to really change his habits, he would need something that was "easy" and "sustainable." Blending gave him that. He started using his blender daily to eat "all the fruits and vegetables you can imagine." Prior to that, he barely ate any vegetables at all, but after a few days, he was surprised to find that he had actually "started to crave those things."

After about a month of using his blender this way, Devin noticed that his body felt different: "I feel healthy. I feel full." Even just the practice of starting his day with a nutrient-rich blend had a noticeable effect: "It makes me want to make good decisions throughout the day."

After feeling the difference that healthy eating can make, Devin was excited to keep up his new habits, especially since "it's so easy and it fits into my life so perfectly."

Once Again, Listen to Your Body

This is such an important topic, we're covering it twice!—earlier, in terms of your physical reaction to foods, and now in terms of your psychological reactions.

Over the years, when talking to patients about what they eat, Dr. Dana has noticed something curious: so many have lost the ability to feel hungry. They have become accustomed to eating on a set schedule of three square meals a day, plus snacks, so they never allow themselves to feel hunger. What's more, what people think of as hunger is often something else, like a desire to feed their feelings or what she calls "mouth-hunger" or cravings, often when they are confronted with the sight or smell of something appetizing. So many of us have become detached from our body's basic hunger cues, the ones telling us when we're running low on fuel.

A growling stomach and lowered energy are generally the first signs of hunger. As your blood sugar drops, signals can progress to headaches, shakiness, and brain fog.

Recall that in our chapter on hydration, we cautioned that you don't want to wait until you feel thirsty to drink water, because by that time, you're already dehydrated. But hunger is different. Our bodies can live much longer without food than they can without water, so hunger cues signal something far less dire. In fact, short periods where we give our bodies time off from eating can have health benefits.

To reacquaint ourselves with feelings of hunger and take advantage of some of the benefits, we suggested you try giving your body a minivacation from eating. By this we mean the practice that's popularly known as *time-restricted eating* (sometimes confused with intermittent fasting, which is when people stop eating for a longer period of time, like a day or more). Time-restricted eating, or what we like to call "taking time off" from eating, means setting aside a period of time overnight when you give your digestive system a rest. It can last anywhere from 10 to 16 hours, and because you will be sleeping for the bulk of that period, it entails extending your noneating window before bedtime and when you first get up in the morning. (See the sidebar for suggestions on how to implement this idea.)

Time-restricted eating is sometimes used as a weight-loss strategy, but that's not why we suggest it here. We think it's worth trying because of the health benefits associated with it. Not only can it help you get in touch with your body's hunger cues, but research suggests that when we give our metabolism a rest, it has a chance to switch gears from processing food to repairing damaged cells and breaking down unwanted chemicals. It's like giving our bodies time to bring in the cleaning crew to tidy everything up. As a result, time-restricted eating may have benefits when it comes to metabolism, obesity prevention, lower incidence of type 2 diabetes, and glycemic control.[5, 6] Some evidence even suggests that it may be protective against cognitive decline and Alzheimer's disease.[7]

Time-restricted eating can also be a good way to break a middle-of-the-night snacking habit. While snacks can certainly be part of any healthy-eating pattern, nighttime snacking is associated with health issues like disrupted sleep, indigestion, and acid reflux.[8]

Give Your Body Some Time Off

Start with 12 Hours: Choose a window of time overnight when you will take time off from eating, keeping in mind that you will be sleeping for the bulk of this period—7 P.M. to 7 A.M., for example. "Time off" applies only to food, so you can still have your morning hydration and black coffee when you wake up, if you like.

Try that for a week or so and if all goes well, extend your time off by an hour. Work your way up to a 16-hour window, if possible. Take note of how you feel at each iteration.

If 12 hours or more feels too long, if you feel overly tired or drained, dial back. Even a 10-hour window can have health benefits.

If this practice leads to excess fatigue or food fixation, stop and return to your regular habits.

Consider Testing Your Reactions

A lot of what we have been talking about here comes down to being mindful about what you eat, why you have chosen it, and how it makes you feel. Once you have built that awareness, it can be enlightening to test whether some of your assumptions about certain foods or ways of eating are actually true. We have encountered a number of people over the years who will say something like, "I hate vegetables" or "I hate fish," even when that's not strictly the case. Maybe they grew up eating overly fishy fish dishes, so they get turned off by the very idea. But then one day, they have fish prepared in a certain way, and they realize that it's possible to like it after all. Many kinds of fresh, white fish, for example, have a mild taste and take on the flavor of what they are cooked with, so the fish-averse might find they like fish in a spicy cioppino or marinated in white wine and cooked on an open grill.

Another example: for a lot of people, salad equals diet food, a plate of bitter greens that ladies eat when they're trying to lose weight. But a foodie friend once pointed out that practically every culture has its salads and that the term can encompass so many different things. The famous encyclopedia of cuisine *Larousse Gastronomique* defines *salad* as: "A dish of raw, cold, or warm cooked foods, usually dressed and seasoned, served as an appetizer, side dish or main course."[9] If you think about it, that can mean practically anything.

We all have certain preferences and opinions about food, both conscious and unconscious, which are sometimes shaped by things other than our taste buds. They can be a result of childhood experiences, cultural perceptions, social influences, and more, which is why it can be useful to test those perceptions once in a while. Do you really "hate salad," or are there some salads you might actually like? What would happen if you thought more broadly about the term? If you're a salad skeptic, consider how many different kinds there are and how they can include far more than just lettuce (or no lettuce at all)—fruits, grains, proteins, and herbs. Think about all the ways different cultures interpret the dish. And then ask yourself: Is there really nothing here that I could like?

WATERMELON FETA SALAD

Watermelon
Feta cheese
Mint leaves
Lemon juice
Olive oil

MEDITERRANEAN TABBOULEH

Bulgur wheat
Parsley
Mint
Cucumber
Onion
Tomato
Olive oil
Lemon or lime juice

WALDORF SALAD

Apples
Grapes
Celery
Toasted walnuts
Greens
Creamy lemony dressing

JAPANESE CUCUMBER SALAD
(*Sunomono*)

Cucumber
Nori
Sesame seeds
Soy sauce
Vinegar

SOUTHWESTERN CHICKEN SALAD

Grilled chicken
Corn
Black Beans
Avocado
Tomatoes
Red onion
Tortilla chips
Lettuce
Spicy lime-cilantro dressing

GREEK SALAD

Olives
Feta cheese
Red onion
Cucumber
Tomato
Oregano
Olive oil

Unleash Your Creativity

In the spirit of playing with your food and trying new things, we want to suggest a few star ingredients that are worth seeking out for your blends. We won't call them *superfoods*, because, as we mentioned before, the term has no official meaning. So, even though it gets thrown around a lot these days, we suggest you take it with a grain of Himalayan pink salt when you hear it.

That said, some ingredients are obviously healthier than others, and we want to suggest some options that are also perhaps a little unusual, which we hope will inspire you to explore and experiment with a wider array of healthy foods. Everything we list here can help you maximize the nutritional value of your meals and increase the diversity in your diet. In the process, you might even find a few new favorites.

In addition to the foods on our list, consider seeking out new ingredients on your own at your local grocery store or farmer's market. If you have a CSA (community-supported agriculture) program near you, that can be a great way to get inspired. Dr. Dana has a subscription to one, and it has introduced her to new greens like mizuna, purslane, and callaloo. She particularly enjoyed discovering sorrel, which has a sweet, lemony flavor and is packed with both vitamin C and vitamin A. Trying new foods can add both flavor and fun to your meals, which can make healthy eating that much more enjoyable. And more enjoyable = more sustainable, which is exactly what we're aiming for.

Aronia Berries: You may not have heard of these, but aronia berries are poised to be the next goji berry or acai because they are a potently rich source of cancer-fighting antioxidants like vitamin C, B vitamins, and various minerals.[10] Also called "chokeberries" because of their sharp taste, some people dislike their flavor when eaten raw, which is why your blender is an asset here. Blending them up with sweeter ingredients will mellow the taste while still allowing you to reap the benefits. They make for a great Enhanced Water flavor or herbal tea—simply add crushed berries to water and let it infuse. You can also mix them in with other berries in any of our Smoothies with Benefits recipes. These may not be available at your local grocery store, but they are easily found either dried or frozen from online retailers.

Cacao Powder: Who doesn't like chocolate? Well, you'll probably like it even better when you find out that it's not only tasty, it can also be really good for you. Rich in a polyphenol called *flavonol*, there's ample research suggesting that cocoa powder and dark chocolate can benefit your cardiovascular health by helping to lower blood pressure and even reduce cholesterol.[11] There are a couple of caveats: we are not talking about cocoa packets here, which often include dairy and sugar. We are talking about 100 percent natural, unsweetened cacao powder, which is sometimes also called cocoa powder. When laden with sugar, chocolate is less healthy, and minimally processed cocoa powder is better for you than commercially processed versions that strip out much of the good stuff your body wants.[12] That's why our recommendation is that you choose natural cocoa rather than alkalized or "dutched" versions. In the U.S., food companies are required to include "processed with alkali" or similar wording on the label. Look for that, often under ingredients, so you know what to avoid.

Enjoy the health (and taste!) benefits of cacao powder in our **Choco-Nutty Tropic** (page 174) smoothie or our **Lovely Lentil Brownie Bites** (page 211).

Sprouts and Microgreens: Sprouts are plants that have just begun to grow after germination. At this early stage, when the plants are still small, they tend to have the highest concentration of nutrients, more so than in their fully matured form. Delicate and often mild in flavor, they typically taste great too, especially to those who shy away from green things. All sorts of plants can be enjoyed in sprout form, including bean sprouts, alfalfa, soy, arugula, clover, wheatgrass, chia, kale, cabbage, broccoli, radish, and more. Microgreens are the next stage of plant growth beyond sprouts, and they, too, are concentrated sources of nutrition—a handful can sometimes equal a whole salad. Uplevel your smoothies or sauces by tossing in either sprouts or microgreens or sprinkle them on top of our **Protein Packed Butternut Squash Soup** (page 197) or our **Enhanced Deviled Eggs** (recipe at the end of this chapter). Both are easy to grow on your kitchen counter (see the Resources section for sources).

Spices: Spices have been prized throughout human history, used not only as seasonings, but also as medicines, currency, and even in religious or ritual offerings. Bundles of dried herbs were hung on doors in medieval Europe, for example, because they were thought to ward off witches![13] We like to think of them more as concentrated flavor and nutrient boosters that you can keep on hand since they have long shelf lives and are often less expensive than fresh ingredients. Play with the following options in your blends or try some of your own.

Cinnamon

Adds a combination of warmth and sweetness.

Known for being rich in antioxidants that may help to control blood sugar.[14]

Blends well with bananas, berries, apples, figs, and cocoa. It also works well to enhance the flavor of meat! Dana often mixes cinnamon into the ground meat filling she uses for stuffed peppers.

Cardamom

Adds a bit of spicy sweetness and a hint of floral.

Known for its phytonutrients, which may have antibacterial and anti-inflammatory benefits.[15]

Blends well with lentils, oranges, dates, and other warm spices like turmeric and cinnamon.

Turmeric

Adds a mild earthy flavor and brilliant color.

Known for potentially helping to reduce inflammation and prevent cancer.[16]

Blends well with carrots, citrus, and ginger. We use it alongside ginger in our **Get Rooted** smoothie (page 180).

Ginger

Adds brightness and zing!

Known for aiding digestion, even used by some for nausea and motion sickness relief.[17]

Blends well with so many things, like squash, carrots, greens, lemon, and peaches. It also makes a delicious, hydrating tea on its own. Just shave some fresh ginger into a mug and pour boiling water over the top.

Make Things Your Own

We have provided you with lots of recipes to try in this book, but because only you know your own body and your own tastes, we also recommend that you learn how to make things your own. With just a little forethought, you can swap out ingredients from our recipes or make your own creations based on what you have on hand, what you feel like in the moment, what tastes good to you, and what's going to fuel your body the best.

As you experiment, remember that blending is a highly forgiving way of preparing food. You can't burn or overcook things—there's no such thing as overblending. You can't undercook things either. The worst that can happen is that your blender has trouble chopping things up, in which case all you have to do is add a bit more liquid and voila! Problem solved.

We have spent a good portion of this book explaining why and how blending can be the cheat you need to achieve good health, but there's another reason too: it's not just good for your health; it's good for the health of the whole planet.

Knowing how to create your own blends is not only a great way to make things taste just the way you like, it's also an effective way to reduce food waste. In the U.S., as much as 40 percent of our food supply never gets eaten,[18] and guess where most of it ends up? In landfills. In fact, food waste is the number one material in our country's landfills. Many people think this is because of waste at farms, food factories, grocery stores, and restaurants, but those aren't the biggest culprits. We are. The biggest source of food waste in this country is our own households.[19] The average American throws out about a pound of food per day.[20]

We wouldn't bother to mention all this if there wasn't something easy and effective you could do about it. Learning how to turn leftover ingredients into sauces, soups, pestos, and smoothies and even how to incorporate things you would otherwise throw out—like beet greens, carrot tops, pumpkin seeds, and soft herb stems—can have a real impact on this issue and provide you with an extra dose of nutrients at the same time. What's more, less food waste also means less stuff to buy during your next trip to the grocery store, which means it's also good for your wallet.

Making things on your own can also help enhance your relationship with food. It will give you a better sense of what you like and what works for your body. And did we mention that it's fun! Experiment and let loose your creativity. The worst that can happen is you make something that doesn't taste great, like when Colin tried sharp-tasting mustard greens in his morning smoothie. He decided they were better for sautéing and has avoided them in his blends ever since. But that's okay. When something like that happens, it just means you get a chance to make something new!

To help with this, we have laid out the building blocks for making your own Smoothie with Benefits, starting from scratch, in the next section. But we hope you won't stop there. We hope you will use these same principles to make your own version of all the recipe categories in this book, from sauces and soups to desserts and even mocktails.

> Try out **"Trash Can" Poaching Sauce** (page 193) that makes use of vegetable scraps that most of us would typically throw away, like carrot tops, broccoli stems, beet greens, and leftover herbs. It's both good for you and good for the environment!

How to Build Your Own Smoothie with Benefits

Use the following formula to create your own fuel-filled smoothie meal that's packed with nutrients, suits your tastes, and will keep you feeling full and energized until lunchtime. This is an important option, because if you like what you're drinking and feel good when you drink it, you're much more likely to stick to the habit!

A well-rounded smoothie meal will fuel your body by providing:

- **Protein:** Protein is a macronutrient that's important for satiety and energy. All our Smoothie with Benefits recipes have around 20 grams of protein, so they can serve as a full meal.

- **Fiber:** Fiber will make you feel fuller longer and is good for maintaining the kind of fertile microbiome that we talked about earlier in this book. Most vegetables and fruits are fiber-rich foods.

- **Healthy Fats:** Fat is another macronutrient that's important for energy production and cellular function, and it plays a key role in the absorption of certain nutrients, like fat-soluble vitamins. Like protein and fiber, it also contributes to satiety. Healthy fats include monounsaturated and polyunsaturated fats, which can be found in nuts, seeds, and plants like avocados and coconut.

- **Micronutrients and Phytonutrients:** Your body requires a wide variety of these for a wide variety of functions. The plants you add to your blend will provide them for you, and the easiest way to cover your bases is to focus on variety: choose both veggies and fruits, change your options from time to time, try different ingredients and color combinations.

Start by Building a Satisfying Base

We like to focus on protein when building our base because our Smoothies with Benefits are meant to serve as full meals. Many of the smoothie recipes you will find online or on social media don't include a full serving of protein, which is a big reason why they don't keep you full for long and serve as more of a snack than a meal.

Protein powder is an option for those who like it for simplicity or are keeping close track of their protein intake for fitness or health reasons. We have included a breakdown of different types of protein powder in the Resources section to help you make informed choices if this is the route you choose to take. However, there are lots of plant proteins to choose from, which, if you know how to use them, can be less expensive, less processed, and tasty options that provide a wide variety of nutrients beyond just protein.

Some options to try:

Nuts: Nuts are an excellent source of protein, fiber, *and* healthy fats, as well as various vitamins and minerals, depending on which ones you choose. In fact, eating nuts may help you live longer (!) as there is a body of research linking them with a reduced risk of heart disease, cancer, and overall mortality.[21] They also happen to be delicious in smoothies and will help make them smooth and creamy. You can try any nut, or blend of nuts, that you like or have on hand, including almonds, Brazil nuts, cashews, chestnuts, hazelnuts, macadamia nuts, peanuts, pecans, pine nuts, pistachios, or walnuts. Or try our Fuel Up Protein Nut Mix, which features equal parts of the following:

- **Almonds** offer about 7 grams of protein per ¼ cup, along with vitamin E, B vitamins, zinc, and iron. They also have among the highest calcium and fiber content of all the nuts.

- **Cashews** offer about 5 grams of protein per ¼ cup and are a great source of B vitamins, potassium, magnesium, zinc, and iron.

- **Walnuts** offer approximately 4.5 grams of protein per ¼ cup and are rich in vitamin E and B vitamins, and they have among the highest level of antioxidants of all the nuts.

Fuel Up Protein Nut Mix

Make ahead your Fuel Up Protein Nut Mix by adding 1 cup each of the following whole nuts to a sealable container. Shake until combined.

Almonds
Cashews
Walnuts

Add ¼ cup of this nut mix to your blend to provide about 6 grams of protein.

Seeds: Like nuts, seeds serve up protein, fiber, healthy fats, and micronutrients, all in one tidy package. You can experiment with chia (white or black), flax, hemp, poppy, pumpkin, sesame, and sunflower. Our seed blend recipe highlights the following trio:

- **Black chia seeds** contain about 4.7 grams of protein per 2-tablespoon serving, along with fiber, calcium, and other trace minerals.

- **Hemp seeds** contain all essential amino acids, making them a complete protein source at 6 grams of protein per 2-tablespoon serving.

- **Flax seeds** contain approximately 5.2 grams of protein per serving alongside fiber and polyphenolic compounds called lignans, which have antioxidant properties and are linked to a reduced risk of heart disease.[22, 23]

Fuel Up Protein Seed Mix

Make ahead your Fuel Up Protein Seed Mix by adding 1 cup each of the following seeds to a sealable container. Shake until combined.

Chia
Hemp
Flax

Add 3 tablespoons of this seed mix to your blend to provide about 7 grams of protein.

Other Smoothie-Friendly Protein Sources

2 tablespoons chia seeds = 4.7 grams

2 tablespoons hemp seeds = 6 grams

2 tablespoons pumpkin seeds = 6 grams

2 tablespoons sunflower seeds = 4 grams

¼ cup almonds = 7 grams

¼ cup walnuts = 4.5 grams

¼ cup pistachios = 6 grams

¼ cup cashew = 5 grams

¼ cup pine nuts = 4.5 grams

2 tablespoons peanut butter = 7 grams

2 tablespoons almond butter = 6.8 grams

½ cup plain Greek yogurt = 12 grams

½ cup plain whole milk yogurt = 4.25 grams

½ cup cottage cheese = 12 grams

½ cup ricotta cheese = 13 grams

¼ cup firm tofu = 10 grams

1 cup edamame = 17 grams

1 cup cooked lentils = 16 grams

1 cup peas = 8 grams

1 cup guava = 4.2 grams

1 cup broccoli = 4 grams

Add Nutrition to Your Base

Next, supercharge your blend with ingredients that will level up its nutrient value and flavor. Draw from the following two categories:

Vegetables: We suggest you include **at least one** veggie in each of your blends. As we've already mentioned, smoothies are a great vehicle for adding extra servings of veggies to your day. Greens like spinach, kale, and Swiss chard blend effortlessly and often tastelessly for those who are greens averse. Zucchini and cauliflower are creative ways of adding texture. Cucumber is refreshing and hydrating. Cooked beets add a bit of sweetness and a gorgeous, deep color. (Be careful: they can also stain your clothes!) Aim for variety and try different combinations from day to day or week to week to highlight different micronutrients and phytonutrients. Veggies will also increase the fiber content of your blends.

Fruit: Fruit is a delightful source of nutrients and flavor. Fruit does have sugar, however, so it's a good idea to be conscious of that fact and not overdo it, especially if you're limiting sugar for health reasons. Even still, in terms of drinking your fruit, blending is better than juicing because it retains all the nutrients of the whole food, including the fiber, which is largely absent from juice. We generally recommend up to **1 cup of fruit**—like berries, grapes, mango or pineapple chunks, peach or nectarine slices—**or ½ cup plus ½ banana** to get the flavor and nutrients you want without an excess of sugar.

Choose Your Liquid

Most smoothies will require **1 cup or so of liquid** per serving to help the ingredients blend up smoothly. That can be anything from simply water (always a healthy choice), to coconut water (for a hit of electrolytes), to milk or milk substitutes (unsweetened versions are the healthiest choice). Leftover Enhanced Water or brewed tea (favorites include hibiscus and licorice, which contains a compound that is 50 times sweeter than sugar) can also lend flavor and a hint of nutrients to your blends. Keep in mind that some liquids will also double as an additional protein source, like the options on the list that follows. (Note: Protein amounts can vary by brand.)

Soy Milk: about 7 to 9 grams per 1 cup

Almond Milk: about 1 to 5 grams per 1 cup

Hemp Milk: about 3 grams per 1 cup

Oat Milk: about 1 to 3 grams per 1 cup

Recipe to Try Today!
Play with a Little Black Dress Recipe

Deviled eggs are one of those versatile, LBD recipes that we talked about earlier, the kind that can serve as a tasty base for adding a whole variety of plants, depending on what you can find at the store, what you already have in your pantry, or what strikes your fancy. We have provided some flavor-enhancing suggestions, but you can also play a little and discover new combinations of your own!

ENHANCED DEVILED EGGS

Makes about 6 servings

6 hard-boiled eggs
½ cup mayo or Greek yogurt
¼ cup whole grain Dijon mustard
1 scallion, bottom removed
2 sprigs fresh dill
8 baby carrots

Peel the hard boiled-eggs and cut them in half. Pop out the yolks and transfer them to a bowl.

Add the mayo or yogurt, mustard, scallion, dill, and carrots to a blender and blend until smooth.

Spoon the mixture into a plastic storage bag and cut off one corner with scissors. Squeeze the yolk mixture into the empty egg whites.

Chill and serve.

Note: Play a little to increase your plant tally by adding things like microgreens, capers, minced bell pepper, or one of the following spice blends to the top of your eggs.

MAKE YOUR OWN SPICE MIXES

Spice up your life by making these tasty and phytonutrient-rich spice mixes. Try adding them not just to your deviled eggs, but also to meats, veggies, soups, scrambled eggs, and even salads. Combine equal amounts of each spice to make the blend.

Mediterranean	Italian	Bay	French	Everything Bagel
sumac	oregano	paprika	thyme	sesame seeds
hyssop	marjoram	celery seed	tarragon	poppy seeds
garlic powder	thyme	red pepper flakes	chervil	garlic powder
rosemary	basil	black pepper	mint	onion powder
fennel seed	sage	mustard seed		salt
thyme	fennel seed			

Cheat Sheet

3 Ways to Play with Your Food . . . Right Away!

- **Pay Attention to How Foods Affect Your Body**
  By trying new things and swapping in or out different ingredients, you can get a better sense of how certain things affect your body. Everyone's body is different, so by being flexible, mindful, and creative, you can find what works best for you.

- **Start Building a More Mindful Relationship with Your Food**
  Rather than always eating based on habit, instinct, or a set schedule, get to know your hunger cues and ask yourself questions about why you make certain choices around food, maybe even challenging your assumptions once in a while about what you like and what you don't. The more we understand why we make certain choices, the easier it is to make ones that leave us feeling nourished.

- **Unleash Your Creativity**
  Preparing meals can be an opportunity to unleash your creativity. Try a new ingredient in your blends or create your own recipes from scratch. Not only does this make meals tastier and more fun, it can also have health benefits!

CHAPTER 6

The 7-Day Beast Blending Lifestyle Plan

It's time to take things to the next level. The plan we are going to walk you through in this chapter brings together all the habits we have been building so far and combines them into a weeklong plan for getting fully fueled so you can unleash the healthy beast inside you—the one who is longing to feel nourished, energized, and satisfied. Those habits include:

- Drinking one blended meal per day from our Smoothies with Benefits program.

- Shifting the balance in your eating pattern to favor more as-nature-intended foods and fewer UPFs.

- Eating a greater variety of plants—more kinds, more colors, and just more overall.

- Being more intentional about getting and staying hydrated.

- Making healthy eating more sustainable by spending some time experimenting, troubleshooting, and playing more with your food.

The goal of this plan is to ground those habits and expand on them to encompass everything you consume in a day, from meals to beverages to snacks and treats. By the end of the week, you will have experienced how "cheating" your way to good health with the help of your blender can become a lifestyle that will sustain you for years to come. You can also return to this plan whenever it feels like you could use some help resetting your habits.

By the end of the week, you will have . . .

- Seen what it's like to nourish yourself without relying on UPFs.

- Reached—even exceeded—your goal of consuming 30 different plants.

- Experienced how easy and delicious healthy eating can be.

- Experienced what it's like to be fully hydrated.

- Noticed how much better these things can make you feel!

The 4 Components of Your Blending Lifestyle Plan

There are four basic parts to this plan that largely mirror what you already consume over the course of a typical day, only with some Fuel Up—style "cheats" to level up the nutrition.

1. Your Smoothie with Benefits Breakfast

Hopefully you have been drinking down your Smoothie with Benefits for breakfast ever since you finished the first chapter. If not, or if not all the time, here's your chance to try the practice for a full week and see how it makes you feel. On the other hand, if you have already been starting your days with a blend, this is a good time to level up. As we explained earlier, the smoothie recipes in this book evolve across three levels to become more veggie-packed and nutrient dense as you go along. Try at least one of our veggie-forward options—or even one of our not-for-the-faint-of-heart options in Level 3!—and take notice of the impact it has on your day.

2. Fuel Up Meals: Lunch and Dinner

We're not asking you to drink all your meals, of course. You're going to want to chew some food too, so, for lunch and dinner, we will provide options that are easy, delicious, and good for you, all at the same time. We are also going to make use of your blender for a lot more than just smoothies. You will whip up simple sauces, condiments, and dressings to uplevel your meals, adding both nutrients *and* flavor.

3. Hydration Breaks: 3 to 4 Times a Day

In Chapter 4, we walked you through a daily schedule that ensures your body gets all the hydration it needs to perform at its best. Too often people underestimate just how important proper hydration is to practically everything our bodies do for us, so we have worked that schedule into your 7-Day Kickstarter Plan. We also offer you a few more hydration options to help you master the habit.

4. Snacks and Desserts: As Desired

This category is optional, of course. Some people just aren't into snacks or treats. Others feel deprived if they don't have them every day. Many of us have one or both on some days and not others, depending on what we're doing, how we're feeling, and how much we've eaten at mealtimes. Wherever you fall on the spectrum, embrace it. Too often people feel shame around snacks and treats, which simply isn't helpful. After all, healthy eating isn't about a single choice. it's about your overall eating pattern. We will show you how these things can be part of a healthy eating pattern and how you can even choose, at time, to uplevel your choices to make them just a little bit healthier but still plenty satisfying and delicious.

Kickstarter Plan Strategies

Before we launch into the plan, let's talk about a few strategies you can use to set yourself up for success.

Master a Few Cooking Techniques

Yes, we're going to ask you to spend some time with a skillet and even turn on your oven once in a while. For some people, this won't be a problem. For others, it will sound like a chore. Before you dismiss the idea out of hand, give us a chance to explain *why* it's worth it to master a few simple cooking techniques and to show you just *how* easy it can be.

First, the *why*: Without question, preparing meals at home makes it easier to eat well. It puts you in control of every element of a dish, of every ingredient you use. This means you can make healthier choices even when you make something that's more of an indulgence. That goes for comfort foods, desserts, snacks, and even cocktails. Not only can you level up the nutrients and level down the less healthy stuff, you can also tailor dishes to suit your tastes for maximum satisfaction.

Research backs up the benefits of cooking. In one large study, eating home-cooked meals was associated with better overall diet quality and a lower likelihood of being overweight or obese. Those who made their own meals more than five times per week also consumed about 2 more ounces of fruits and nearly 3.5 more ounces of veggies every day.[1] In other words, they naturally ate more plants, which, as you already know, is key to good health.

Now, for the *how*: we're going to introduce you to our simple cooking techniques, which anyone of any skill level can master. They include four delicious yet straightforward ways to cook healthy proteins that you can build your meals around, including:

- Simple Roasted Chicken
- Simple Grilled or Broiled Steak
- Simple Poached Salmon
- Simple Vegan Mushroom Burger

For your plan this week, we suggest you start with the chicken. After all, it's easy, cost-effective, versatile, *and* tasty—and we're going to show you how you can use one roast chicken to make a variety of healthy dishes. (If you're a vegetarian or pescatarian, or if you're one of the few people out there who doesn't like chicken, you're welcome to choose one of the other options, of course.) The only potential drawback to roasting a chicken is that it takes time, but that won't be a problem if you plan ahead, which is the next strategy we're going to talk about.

Planning Ahead Is Key

Let's face it: there are going to be times when eating well feels like a lot to manage. When you're tired, stressed, grumpy, or short on time, it's easy to reach for something that's satisfying in the short term but provides inferior fuel in the long run. One of the most effective ways to promote healthier eating is to decide what you're going to eat *before* you're hungry. That means not only having a meal plan in mind, but also strategizing about what snacks and treats you will have at the ready so that you have some healthy/healthier options to choose from when the mood strikes.

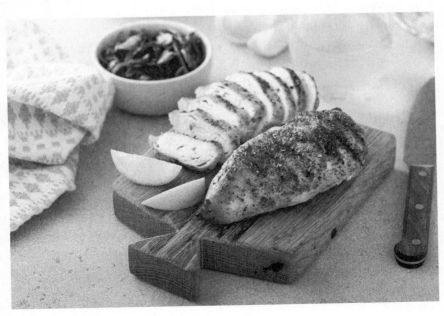

PLAN AHEAD:
Lunches and Dinners

We will provide you with recipes in the coming pages, but it's also a good idea to get into the habit of building your own healthy meals. For either lunch or dinner, use the following formula to help you envision how to fill your plate:

1 Protein + Unlimited Veggies + 1 Optional Side

Paired with

1 Blended Enhancement (Optional but Encouraged)

= a Fuel Up Meal

Proteins can be meats, seafood, eggs, or vegetarian proteins like tofu, lentils, or beans (which also count toward your plant tally!). When it comes to cooking methods, your protein can be baked, grilled, roasted, sautéed, poached, stir-fried, air-fried, or thrown into a pressure cooker. The only method we recommend against is deep frying. Because fried foods can take a real toll on your health,[2] we hope you will consider them an occasional indulgence in general and avoid them for the duration of this plan. In terms of portions, a good rule of thumb is that one serving is about the size of the palm of your hand. Of course, that's a very general rule, and you will have to adjust according to your appetite and activity level.

Veggies can be literally anything in this category. Again, just about any cooking method besides deep frying works great, or you can enjoy them raw. As you already know, very few of us are eating the recommended amount of vegetables, and this is your chance to play a little, experiment, and find some new options that you like. We recommend at least two different types of veggies per meal, with no upward limit!

Optional Sides can be any whole grain, including quinoa, farro, barley, brown rice, or wild rice. They can also be something like beans, lentils, or sliced avocado. Of course, you may not need a side dish if you opt for something like a stew, a soup, or a protein-rich salad. Choose what works for you.

Blended Enhancements are things like sauces, marinades, dressings, and dips that will uplevel your nutrition and make your dishes more flavorful and fun, all at the same time. This is also a great opportunity to swap out some of the UPFs in your diet by making healthier versions of your favorite packaged foods at home. And it's a fantastic way to stretch your budget, since many leftover ingredients, like herbs and veggies, can be repurposed to make delicious meal enhancements for use throughout the week. Of course, you don't need a blended enhancement with every meal, but over the course of this week, we're going to ask you to try a few to experience how they can enhance your meals.

PLAN AHEAD:
Snacks and Desserts

Snacks: Consider what you typically reach for and use some of the swapping strategies we talked about in Chapter 2 to uplevel them. If you like something salty like potato chips, look for a healthier substitute like salted nuts. If you often get a sweet tooth in the afternoon, have some fruit on hand or try one of the snack smoothies you will find in the plan or even one of our sweeter Salad Shooters (**Feel the Beet** on page 202 is one of the sweeter options). Make sure to have the options ready, meaning if you're opting for crudités with our Enhanced Ranch Dressing for your afternoon snack, have the dressing made and the veggies chopped and ready. Prepping things ahead makes it that much easier to choose the healthier option.

Desserts: The same swapping strategy can work for treats, and we offer some healthy-delicious recipes and quick-grab options in the plan that will help you satisfy your sweet tooth without feeling deprived. It's a good idea to have some healthier options ready *before* the cravings start. (We recommend our decadent **Lovely Lentil Brownie Bites** on page 211, for example.) However, when nothing but an Entenmann's brownie will do, eat the brownie and don't beat yourself up. When we make these choices, let's allow ourselves to enjoy them—that's the healthiest outlook any of us can have.

Your 7-Day Blending Lifestyle Plan Prep

1. **Choose Your Meals.** Consult the "day in the life" schedule and recipes that start on page 145 and choose what you will make for the week in each of the four categories: your Smoothie with Benefits Breakfast, Fuel Up Meals, Infused Hydration, and Snacks and Desserts. Fill them in on the Meal Chart below.

2. **Create Your Shopping List.** Use this chart to create a grocery list for the week. In addition to the ingredients needed to make your meals, remember to include some healthy, quick-grab snack and dessert options to have on hand. You will find a list of suggestions in the plan.

3. **Make-Ahead Items.** We recommend you cook a few things in advance to get a jump start on the week. We have made a few suggestions to get you started, but feel free to swap in any of the options from the recipe chapter that follows if there's something that suits you better.

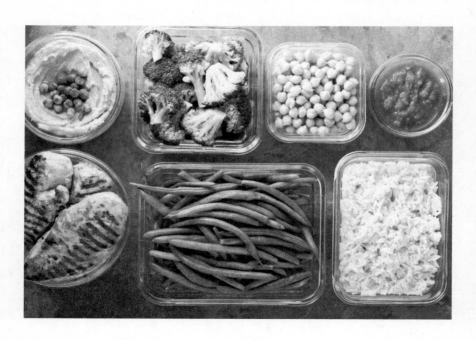

7-Day Meal Chart

Fill in the chart using our recipes or by making your own dishes using our Fuel Up Meal formula. We got you started by suggesting a few make-ahead items (a roasted chicken, a salad dressing, and a sauce) that you can use in multiple ways throughout the week.

	Breakfast Blends	Fuel Up Lunch	Fuel Up Dinner	Snack & Dessert Options (if desired)
Saturday			Simple Roasted Chicken with Seasoned Veggies	Crudités with Enhanced Ranch Dressing
Sunday		Green Salad with Enhanced Ranch Dressing Topped with Protein of Your Choice	Chicken, Shrimp, or Tofu Stir-Fry with Tangy Cilantro Citrus Sauce	
Monday		Dana's Herbaceous Chicken Salad Wrap		
Tuesday				
Wednesday				
Thursday				
Friday				

Recommended Make-Ahead Items to Kick Things Off Right!

✓ Choose a simple protein recipe to make. We recommend our **Simple Roasted Chicken with Seasoned Veggies** (page 154).

✓ Choose a nutrient-dense salad dressing to make, which can be used in multiple recipes. We commend our **Enhanced Ranch Dressing** to use on salads and as a snack dip.

✓ Choose a healthy and flavorful sauce, which can be used in multiple recipes. We recommend our **Tangy Cilantro Citrus Sauce** (page 184) to use as a stir-fry sauce and to dress veggies.

Quick Tips

• Cook meals that will leave you with leftovers for additional meals and even snacks.

• Make sure you have a couple quick-turnaround options for busy days. Eggs, tofu, cooked shrimp, and other precooked proteins are good bets.

• Pick things that sound good! Eating well shouldn't feel like deprivation.

The 7-Day Beast Blending Lifestyle Plan

A Day in the Life

Time to get started! The following pages will walk you through each element of Beast Blending Lifestyle eating and hydration plan. It includes directions, meal suggestions, and recipes. See Chapter 7 for additional recipes if some of our recommendations don't work for you.

Morning Hydration

Start your day with a large glass of water

Hot or cold; plain or with a pinch of salt, squeeze of lemon, or other natural flavoring like sliced cucumber, strawberries, mint leaves, or whatever else sounds good. Coffee or tea can follow.

Smoothie with Benefits Breakfast

Choose one per day

You can try 7 different smoothies for each day of the week or repeat a recipe if you want to use up ingredients or have a favorite. We encourage you to **try at least 3 options during the week** so you can maximize the variety of plants and nutrients that you consume. We also encourage you to try at least one veggie-forward option from either Level 2 or 3. Recipes start on page 173.

Midmorning Hydration and Snack Break

Snacks are always optional and completely up to you. If you feel like you want something, try one of the healthy choices below. Hydration, on the other hand, is strongly encouraged! Try one of our Enhanced Water options, or, in a pinch, a plain glass of water will do.

Hydration Options

Herbal tea, hot or cold

Any of our Enhanced Water Infusions (starting on page 212)

Any of our Hydration Blends like one of our make-your-own electrolyte water recipes (starting on page 215)

Water with cut-up fruit or other flavorings like berries, cucumber, ginger, or mint

Water with a pinch of salt

Just plain water

Snack Options

Crudités with one of our hummus recipes or our Enhanced Ranch Dressing

A mugful of warm vegetable or bone broth, or one of our Enhanced Broths (starting on page 192)

A handful of nuts like almonds or pecans, or try mixed nuts to increase your plant tally

Apple slices with nut butter

A hard-boiled egg

Leftovers! A few bites of last night's dinner can make a satisfying snack, and it's a great way to avoid wasting food

Fuel Up Lunch

Create Your Own Meals Using Our Formula:

1 Protein + Unlimited Veggies + 1 Optional Side
Paired with
1 Blended Enhancement (Optional but Encouraged)
= Fuel Up Lunch

Or, Choose from the Fuel Up Meal Ideas Below.
(Feel free to use any of our dinner ideas for lunch,
or our simple cooking techniques on page 154.)

Lunch Ideas

Dana's Herbaceous Chicken Salad Wrap (page 161)

Mediterranean Rotisserie Tacos (page 164)

Tuna Romaine Boats (page 162)

Salad topped with a burger or salmon

Simple Vegan Mushroom Burger (page 158)

Last night's leftovers

Midday Hydration and Snack Break

For your afternoon break, you're welcome to choose any of the structured water or snack options listed above. Or try one of the snack smoothies below. These are different from our breakfast blends because they're smaller portions, lighter (lower in protein), and not meant to serve as a full meal.

GINGER ZINGER SNACK SMOOTHIE

1 cup water
1 cup spinach
1 green apple, cored and seeded
1-inch chunk of ginger
1 tablespoon chia seeds
½ cup ice (optional)

TROPICAL MANGO SNACK SMOOTHIE

1 cup water
1 cup fresh kale
1 cup frozen mango chunks
1 cup frozen pineapple chunks
1 tablespoon chia seed
½ cup ice (optional)

Fuel Up Dinner

Create Your Own Meals
Using Our Formula:

1 Protein + Unlimited Veggies + 1 Optional Side
Paired with
1 Blended Enhancement (Optional but Encouraged)
= Fuel Up Dinner
Or, Choose from the Fuel Up Meal Ideas Below.
(Feel free to use any of our lunch ideas for dinner,
or our simple cooking techniques on page 154.)

Dinner Ideas

Simple Roasted Chicken with Seasoned Veggies (page 154)

Roasted Cauliflower Steaks with Zesty Walnut Pesto
(page 166)

Simple Poached Salmon with wild rice or green salad
(page 156)

Simple Grilled Steak with Superb Steak Sauce and
a mixed veggie sauté (page 157)

Beef with Peppers and Onions (page 165)

Shrimp, Tofu, or Chicken Stir-Fry with an Enhanced Stir-Fry
Sauce (page 168)

Dessert Time

Everything you eat doesn't have to be all good for you, all the time. By the same token, just because something is labeled a "dessert" doesn't mean it has to be all bad for you either. The Sweets and Treats section of our recipe chapter has a range of options, from puddings to frozen desserts to baked goods like brownies and mini muffins, each with its own twist that will help you indulge in a way that's just a little bit healthier. We are also providing you with some quick-grab options for when you haven't made something ahead of time.

Quick Dessert Options

Frozen grapes

Fresh fruit

A dessert smoothie like our **"Nice" Cream Smoothie** or **Colin's Date Night Smoothie** (page 207)

Of course, you don't have to have dessert if you don't want to. Instead, or in addition, this might be a good chance to hydrate one last time. Just make sure to consider whether doing so will cause you to have to use the bathroom during the night. If nighttime urination is a problem, try cutting off liquids an hour or more before bedtime and remind yourself to use the bathroom just before sleep.

End-of-the-Week
Questions to Ask Yourself

✓ How many plants were you able to consume this week? If you are like most home cooks, it was more than usual!

✓ How did this way of eating make you feel? The goal is to feel healthier, happier, more vibrant, and full of energy, all at once.

✓ What, if anything, was difficult for you? What might become difficult if you continued the plan beyond this one week?

✓ What tweaks could you make to this plan to make it more sustainable for you? Consult Chapter 6 for troubleshooting suggestions.

Case Study: Amy

A marketing professional in her late 30s, Amy had been on and off diets most of her adult life. As a busy career woman, she naturally gravitated toward quick, processed foods, which she knew weren't all that good for her. So, in an effort to get healthier, she would periodically try another diet.

Amy had attempted a lot of different eating programs and cleanses over the years. She felt like she had been able to make some small improvements to the way she ate, but she was still a regular soda drinker, a habit she was looking to curb, and she wasn't eating a lot of fruits and vegetables. When it came to produce in particular, the thought of consuming more of those nutrient-rich foods made her feel overwhelmed. "I tried to get them in. I knew it was important," she said. But, because she didn't really know how to prepare them, she often ate them raw, which just didn't taste good to her. Soon she would go back to her processed favorites.

That is, until she tried our Beast Blending Lifestyle Plan. "I was so excited for all the recipes, for the smoothies, to have all of those options in the morning," she explained. And then, "having flexibility throughout the rest of the day" made a real difference. "A lot of the eating programs I followed in the past were really strict, but this one wasn't," Amy added. Plus, drinking infused water throughout the day helped her reduce the amount of soda she was drinking.

"I noticed over time how my energy was getting better and better, and my sleep started to get better. My bowel movements started to be more regular overall. I felt really good inside." Those are the feelings that inspired Amy to keep the plan going beyond seven days for a full four weeks.

"This was the first time I was excited about an eating plan, because I felt empowered," Amy told us. "It's amazing for me to think how natural it now is to make sure I have vegetables at every meal. And the smoothie in the morning really sets my day up for success . . .

"I just assumed, like every other eating plan, the second I was done, I would immediately run for pizza, but it's been completely different and I'm so grateful." What made it last? Amy attributed it to how the plan made her feel: "I feel so good and want to continue feeling good. I want to continue this feeling of health and energy."

Lifestyle Plan Cooking Recipes

In the next chapter, you will find a wide variety of blended recipes for your smoothies, sauces, dressings, soups, desserts, and more. What follows are cooking recipes that don't necessarily require your blender. Remember, we do not intend for you to blend all your food! It's important to chew some too, and the recipes in the following pages will help fill in those gaps during your weeklong plan. Feel free to also concoct meals of your own using our Fuel Up Meal Formula. Some basic protein and veggie preparation recipes are included to help you build them.

We have included far more recipes here than you will need for a single week, but we wanted to provide you with a range of options to ensure you will find plenty of things to enjoy! You might also consider extending this plan beyond 7 days so you can try more recipes. Our hope is that you will even consider extending it indefinitely and make it a way of life!

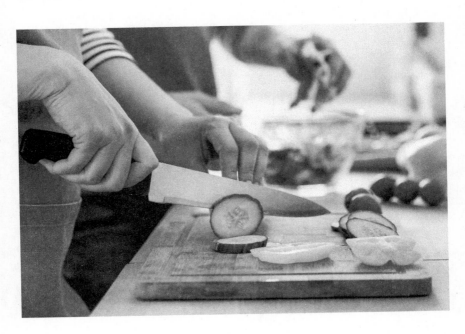

Simple Protein Cooking Techniques

Makes about 4 servings

- 3-pound whole chicken
- 2 tablespoons olive oil, divided
- Salt and pepper to taste
- Pinch garlic powder
- 2 stalks celery, diced
- 2 large carrots, diced
- 1 cup sliced mushrooms
- 1 large yellow onion, diced
- A few sprigs of herbs like rosemary and/or thyme

Preheat the oven to 350 degrees Fahrenheit.

Remove anything from inside the whole chicken. Dry the chicken skin with a paper towel.

Massage the outside of the chicken with a tablespoon of olive oil. Season with salt, pepper, and garlic powder.

Add the remaining olive oil to the pan.

Fill the cavity with celery, carrots, mushrooms, onion, and herbs. If there are extra vegetables, just toss them in the bottom of the pan to roast.

Place chicken in a roasting pan or on a baking sheet with a rack.

Cook for about 1 hour and 30 minutes or until the thickest part of the chicken reaches 165 degrees Fahrenheit.

Remove the vegetables from the inside of the chicken and serve as a side dish with or without rice.

Note: Consider picking the leftover chicken and using it to make a chicken stir-fry with one of our enhanced sauces and/or Dana's Herbaceous Chicken Salad (page 161).

Chicken Cheats

☀ If you're cooking for more than just yourself, consider roasting two chickens at once so you have enough for everyone, plus leftovers (for the whole family, including the dog!).

☀ If you really don't want to cook, buy a rotisserie chicken (or two) at your local grocery store. It will work just as well in the recipes provided.

SIMPLE POACHED SALMON

Makes about 2 to 3 servings

1 cup "Trash Can" Poaching Broth (page 193) or vegetable broth
½ yellow onion, diced
1 teaspoon lemon zest
Pinch sea salt
1 pound wild salmon filets

Heat poaching sauce or veggie broth in a small skillet over medium heat.

Add onion, lemon zest, and sea salt to the water and let simmer for about 5 minutes, until just before boiling.

Gently place the salmon into the liquid so it's almost covered.

Cover with a lid and cook for about 8 to 10 minutes, depending on how you like it. Fish is perfectly cooked when it reaches 140 degrees Fahrenheit.

Squeeze lemon juice over your fish and add fresh herbs, if you like.

Enjoy right away with wild rice or salad.

Note: This recipe is so easy and forgiving. It also works well with other kinds of fish like sea bass, cod, halibut, you name it! Leftovers will last in the fridge for 3 days.

SIMPLE GRILLED OR BROILED STEAK

Makes 4 servings

4½-inch-thick New York strip steaks	Sea salt and pepper to taste
4 sprigs fresh rosemary	Pinch garlic powder

Remove steaks from the refrigerator about 20 minutes before grilling.

Turn your grill on at a high temperature, about 500 degrees Fahrenheit, and keep it covered.

Rub each piece of steak with the rosemary sprigs for flavor.

Season both sides of the steaks with a light dusting of pepper and garlic powder. It's okay to be generous with the salt.

Place steaks on the grill and leave the lid open while they cook. Add 2 rosemary sprigs to the top of each steak.

Cook for about 3 minutes and then rotate a quarter turn to create grill marks. Cook for about 3 minutes more.

Flip steaks and cook for another 3 to 5 minutes depending on desired level of doneness (see note), moving rosemary to the top side. Rotate a quarter turn about halfway through to create grill marks. If steaks are burning, move them to a cooler section of the grill to finish cooking.

To broil in oven:

Make sure the oven rack is at least 4 inches from the broiler and preheat the broiler.

Season steak the same way as you would for grilling.

Spray a baking sheet with a bit of olive or avocado oil.

Add steaks to the baking sheet and place into the broiler. Add rosemary to the top.

Cook for about 4 minutes. Flip the steaks and cook for another 3 minutes or until desired temperature is reached. Keep a close eye while cooking, as steaks can burn quickly under the broiler.

Note: The best way to tell when steaks are done is to use an instant-read thermometer. Remove steaks just before desired temperature is achieved and let them rest before serving:

Rare = 120 degrees • Medium rare = 130 degrees • Medium = 140 degrees
Medium well = 150 degrees • Well done = 160 degrees

SIMPLE VEGAN MUSHROOM BURGERS (or Balls)

Makes about 4 servings

½ cup walnuts

2 cloves garlic

¼ cup hemp seed

½ cup flax seed

1 tablespoon olive oil

3 cups diced portobello mushrooms

½ yellow onion, diced

1 tablespoon Worcestershire sauce

1 capful liquid smoke (optional)

2 cups cooked brown rice, freshly cooked

½ cup aquafaba*

Blend walnut, garlic, and hemp and flax seed into a textured paste.

In a saucepan, heat olive oil. Add in diced mushroom and onion. Sauté until onions are lightly browned.

Add in walnut paste, Worcestershire sauce, and liquid smoke (if using) and continue to sauté the mixture until soft.

Transfer the mixture to a bowl. Fold in the rice and stir until well combined.

Pour in aquafaba and let sit until the mixture is still warm but comfortable to handle.

Form into medium-sized balls or patties and place on a wax paper–lined cookie sheet. (Tip: Wiping hands after shaping each one makes it easier to create balls and patties.)

Bake at 425°F for 10 minutes, then flip burgers or roll meatballs over and bake for another 10 minutes. (Or air-fry for about 15 minutes.)

Dress just as you would any burger.

Our **Superb Steak Sauce** (page 60) or **Don't Mess with Texas BBQ Sauce** (page 190) are great choices for upleveling the nutrition and the flavor of these burgers. Or enjoy meatball or falafel-style in a lettuce wrap or on top of a salad.

* *Aquafaba* is the liquid from a can of chickpeas. (Yes, it has a name!) Alternatively, you can use the liquid from any mild-tasting bean, or use 2 eggs instead for a nonvegan, higher-protein version.

Quick and Easy
Veggie Prep Ideas

BAKED OR MASHED SWEET POTATOES

To bake:

Stab the potatoes with a fork a few times.

Bake them at 375 degrees Fahrenheit for about 45 minutes, or until it's easy to poke a fork into them.

To mash:

Peel and cube the sweet potatoes and boil them in water until tender.

Add a splash or 2 of almond milk, a pat of butter, and salt to taste.

Mash until you achieve the desired texture.

MIXED VEGGIE SAUTÉ

Heat a tablespoon of olive oil in a pan over medium heat.

Sauté a clove of chopped, fresh garlic until it's fragrant and just starting to brown.

Add whatever chopped veggies you have on hand, like bell peppers, carrots, bok choy, and/or green beans and sauté them until tender.

Salt and pepper to taste.

SIMPLE BRUSSELS SPROUTS

To air-fry:

1. Toss halved Brussels sprouts in a bit of olive oil to coat.

2. Salt and pepper to taste.

3. Air-fry the sprouts at 350 degrees Fahrenheit for 8 to 10 minutes, or until tender.

To braise:

Heat a tablespoon of olive oil in a pan over medium heat.

Add halved Brussels sprouts, flat side down, and sauté for about 3 minutes.

Add 2 to 3 tablespoons of water, give a quick stir, and cover for 3 to 4 minutes.

Remove lid, stir, and continue to sauté until the water cooks off and the sprouts are tender.

Note: The above braising technique also works well with green beans.

STEAMED VEGETABLES

Using a steamer pot with a basket, fill the bottom of the pot with about an inch of water and bring it to a boil over medium-high heat.

Insert the basket and fill with veggies of your choice, like bok choy, broccoli, or spinach. Season with salt to taste.

Cover and cook until veggies are tender, typically 5 to 10 minutes, depending on the size of your veggies.

Lunch and Dinner Options

DANA'S HERBACEOUS CHICKEN SALAD

Makes about 4 servings

4 cups chopped cooked chicken or leftover rotisserie chicken
½ cup chopped walnuts or almonds
½ cup chopped apple or grapes
1 cup Greek yogurt
¼ cup chopped parsley
¼ cup chopped dill
2 teaspoons whole grain Dijon mustard
Juice of 1 lemon
Salt and pepper to taste

Add chopped chicken, nuts, and chopped apple to a large bowl.

Add the yogurt, herbs, mustard, and lemon juice to a blender cup and pulse until well blended but still textured.

Pour the blended yogurt mixture over the chicken, nuts, and apple. Stir until all of the ingredients are combined.

Chill for 1 hour (if you can wait. If not . . . dig in).

Salt and pepper to taste and serve on top of a green salad or in our Spinach Wraps or Red Lentil Wraps (pages 222 and 223).

Note: Leftovers last in the fridge for about 3 days.

TUNA ROMAINE BOATS

Makes about 2 servings

One 5-ounce can tuna in water, drained
¼ white onion and/or apple, diced (if raw onion is not your thing)
½ stalk celery, diced
Fresh or dried dill to taste (optional)
2 tablespoons Greek yogurt
4 large, sturdy romaine leaves

Place all ingredients except romaine leaves in a bowl and mix well.

Place the romaine leaves spine side down on a plate and fill with tuna mixture.

Salt and pepper to taste.

Note: You can add shaved carrot, tomato, microgreens, capers, or any veggie that sounds good to the top to keep things interesting. Or, Dana's favorite simplified version is to add a cup of prepared broccoli slaw (broccoli, carrots, and purple cabbage) to the tuna along with the Greek yogurt. Mix well and you're done!

GRILLED LEMON PEPPER CHICKEN

Makes about 2 servings

2 chicken breasts
Juice of 1 lemon
1 pinch ground black pepper
1 pinch sea salt
1 tablespoon olive oil

Slice chicken breasts in half lengthwise so you have several thinner breasts.

Marinate breasts in the lemon juice for 20 minutes and sprinkle them with salt and pepper.

Either grill, broil, or pan-fry the breasts (with a little olive oil in the pan) until thoroughly cooked.

Note: As long as you eat your chicken within 3 days, you can use it in a ton of different ways.

Ways to serve:

Hot with a side of brown rice and sautéed green beans or cut up and add to the top of a salad with black beans and a dollop of hummus.

Make a veggie stir-fry and throw in a serving of chicken for a delicious meal.

QUICK AND DELICIOUS SLOW COOKER SALSA CHICKEN

Makes about 6 servings

1 tablespoon olive oil
4 skinless chicken breasts
2 cups Did Someone Say Salsa? (page 200)
1 large zucchini, cut into ¼-inch cubes
1 cup sliced white mushroom
1 bell pepper, diced
1 white onion, diced
1 cup Veggie Strong Broth Blend (page 192)
Salt and pepper to taste

Add olive oil to the bottom of the crockpot, and then add the remaining ingredients. Set the pot on low and cook for 6+ hours.

Serve the salsa chicken over rice and/or with diced avocado on top.

MEDITERRANEAN ROTISSERIE TACOS

Makes about 1 serving

2 Red Lentil Wraps (page 223) or tortillas
2 tablespoons hummus (page 198)
1 cup rotisserie or leftover chicken, shredded or cubed
¼ cucumber, diced
1 Roma tomato, diced

Warm up the wraps or tortillas on very low heat on the stovetop. (Keep flipping or they will burn!)

Add 1 tablespoon hummus to each tortilla.

Add ½ cup of chicken to each tortilla and top with cucumber and tomato.

Fold each tortilla into a taco shape and enjoy!

Note: You can also top with microgreens, shaved carrot, and/or red onion if you want to get in more plant servings.

BEEF WITH PEPPERS AND ONIONS

Makes about 4 servings

1 pound lean beef (top sirloin is a good choice)
1 pinch sea salt
1 teaspoon ground black pepper
1 tablespoon olive oil
2 cloves garlic, thinly sliced
1 bell pepper, sliced
1 yellow onion, sliced

Chop up beef into bite-sized chunks and season with salt and pepper.

Heat a skillet over medium heat and add olive oil. Add garlic and cook until fragrant, about 30 seconds.

Add beef and stir a few times to cook evenly.

After about 5 minutes, add the peppers and onions.

Cook until the onion is translucent and peppers are tender yet crisp. Serve over rice, in a wrap, or with a side vegetable.

Note: Eat or freeze within 3 days.

ROASTED CAULIFLOWER STEAKS
with Zesty Walnut Pesto

Makes about 4 servings

1 head cauliflower
⅓ cup unsalted walnuts
½ cup extra virgin olive oil, divided, plus more as needed
1 bunch fresh cilantro or parsley leaves
2 cloves garlic
1 jalapeño pepper, stemmed, seeded (optional)
3 tablespoons shredded Parmesan cheese
Juice of ½ lime
½ teaspoon ground cumin
Salt and pepper to taste

Preheat oven to 400°F.

Slice the cauliflower into ½-inch thick steaks and set aside. (The edges will crumble a bit, so season and roast the crumbs too!)

In a dry pan, toast walnuts over medium-low heat for several minutes until fragrant and slightly brown. Shake the pan occasionally and keep a close eye on them, because they can burn quickly.

In a blender, combine all remaining ingredients except salt and pepper, and pulse several times until the pesto is well combined but still slightly textured. Add salt and pepper to taste.

Line a baking sheet (or two if needed) with parchment paper and oil it lightly. Using a basting brush, spread a bit of pesto on the top side of the steaks and place in the oven.

Flip the cauliflower steaks after about 10 minutes and baste the top side again. Cook until golden brown on the edges and tender. (Use a fork or toothpick to check tenderness.)

Move the cauliflower steaks to plates and top with additional pesto. Salt and pepper to taste.

Note: Tastes great with hummus. Leftovers last for 3 days in the fridge, and leftover toasted walnuts make a great topping for salads.

SHRIMP STIR-FRY
with Enhanced Stir-Fry Sauce

Makes about 4 servings

2 tablespoons olive or sesame oil
1 bell pepper, sliced
2 medium carrots, sliced
1 red onion, sliced
1 cup chopped green beans
1 head bok choy, chopped
1 pound medium-sized shrimp, peeled and deveined
1 pinch sea salt
1 teaspoon ground black pepper
¼ cup Enhanced Stir-Fry Sauce (page 184)

Heat a skillet over medium heat and add oil.

Add veggies, bok choy last, and cook until almost tender. Toss in the shrimp, season them with salt and pepper, and cook until they turn pink.

Add Enhanced Stir-Fry Sauce and stir to combine.

Serve over brown rice.

Note: This makes for great leftovers to eat either hot or cold. Eat or freeze within 3 days. Chunks of chicken or extra-firm tofu also work well in place of shrimp.

CHICKEN STIR-FRY
with Tangy Cilantro Citrus Sauce

Makes about 2 servings

2 tablespoons olive or sesame oil

1 pound boneless, skinless chicken breast, cubed

2 medium-sized carrots, sliced

2 celery stalks, sliced

1 small broccoli head, stemmed and chopped

1 small white onion, sliced

½ cup Tangy Cilantro Citrus Sauce (page 184)

Heat skillet over medium heat and add oil. Add chicken and cook for about 5 minutes.

Add the vegetables and Tangy Cilantro Citrus Sauce and stir-fry until the vegetables are tender.

Serve over brown or white rice.

Note: This makes for great leftovers to eat either hot or cold. Eat or freeze within 3 days. Chunks of hard tofu or shrimp also work well in place of chicken.

HENRY'S STUFFED PEPPERS

Makes about 4 servings

2 tablespoons olive oil
1 large zucchini, cut into ¼-inch cubes
1 small yellow onion, diced
2 cloves garlic, minced
1 pound ground beef or turkey
One 6-ounce can tomato paste
¼ teaspoon cinnamon
¼ teaspoon turmeric
Salt and pepper to taste
4 large green bell peppers
Grated Parmesan cheese (optional)

Preheat oven to 350°F.

Heat a large skillet over medium heat and add olive oil. Add zucchini, onions, and garlic and cook until onions are translucent.

Add ground meat and cook, stirring occasionally, until browned.

Add tomato paste and spices and stir to combine. Season with salt and pepper to taste and let the mixture simmer until flavors combine, about 5 minutes.

In a separate pot, boil water. Cut the tops off the peppers and seed them. (Use the tops in your salad.)

Place the cleaned peppers in the boiling water and let them soften, about 6 minutes. (You will need to use a spoon to push the peppers so they fill up with water and can cook.)

Use tongs to remove the peppers, shaking out excess water, and place them on a baking sheet with sides.

Spoon the meat mixture into the peppers, filling them to the top. Sprinkle them heavily with grated cheese, if desired.

Cover the peppers with foil and bake for 20 minutes.

Blends with Benefits Recipes

Measurement Cheat

Blending is a very flexible and forgiving way to prepare food. So, if you are more of an intuitive cook or feel like it's too much trouble to get out and then clean your measuring cups and spoons, you can improvise. Measure ingredients once and then use the palm of your hand as a guide. What does a tablespoon of dried herbs versus a teaspoon look like in your palm, for example? In our estimation, a cup works out to be about a handful and ⅛ teaspoon is about a pinch, but you can adjust accordingly. This cheat will work with practically all the recipes in this chapter, with the exception of the baked treats in our dessert section.

Smoothies with Benefits

Our smoothie recipes are unique in a couple of ways. First, they are designed to serve as full meals containing protein, healthy fats, fiber, and at least one serving of the fruits and vegetables that most of us aren't getting enough of.

Second, they aren't just one-off recipes. We have created an entire Smoothies with Benefits Program with three levels that can help your tastes evolve in a healthier direction.

- Level 1 recipes are sweeter and more fruit-forward.

- Level 2 recipes are more vegetable-forward with more complex flavor profiles.

- Level 3 includes not-for-the-faint-of-heart options that are packed with nutrients.

All our recipes are good for you, but some pack in more nutritional benefits than others, which is why our Smoothie with Benefits Program offers you different levels to try. Our intention is for you to eat as healthfully as possible within the context of what works for you. These levels should help you find a balance between what's good for you and what tastes good to you, because both are important.

Directions for Making Smoothies with Benefits

1. Add all ingredients to your blender.

2. Blend until smooth, about 1 minute.

3. Enjoy!

All recipes make about 1 serving.

Note: You can use fresh or frozen versions of any of the fruits and vegetables listed in these recipes. However, if you use only fresh, make sure to include ice. This is because a blender creates a bit of heat when it's working, and most of us like our smoothies cold!

Level 1:
Starter Smoothies

CHOCO-NUTTY TROPIC

1 cup unsweetened nut, seed, or oat milk
¼ cup Fuel Up Protein Nut Mix (see page 129) or cashews
½ cup pineapple chunks
1 cup baby spinach
1 cup peas (frozen recommended)
½ banana
1 tablespoon cacao powder
½ cup ice cubes (optional)

CHERRY BERRY SEEDY

1 cup unsweetened nut, seed, or oat milk
¼ cup Fuel Up Protein Seed Mix (see page130) or hemp seeds
¼ cup Fuel Up Protein Nut Mix (see page 129) or almonds
2 tablespoons raspberries or dried aronia berries
½ cup pitted cherries
1 cup baby spinach
½ banana
½ cup ice cubes (optional)

QUICK AND TASTY

1 cup unsweetened nut, seed, or oat milk
½ banana
1 cup mixed berries
1 cup mixed leafy greens
1 serving protein powder
½ cup ice cubes (optional)

WILD FOR WALNUTS

1 cup unsweetened nut, seed, or oat milk
¼ cup walnuts or Fuel Up Protein Nut Mix (see page 129)
2 cups baby spinach
½ cup pineapple chunks
½ cup pitted cherries
1 serving protein powder
1 pinch ground cinnamon
½ cup ice cubes (optional)

Level 2:
Step Up Your Smoothie Game

MICRO MAMMA BLEND

1 cup unsweetened almond or coconut milk
2 cups mixed greens
1 medium carrot, chopped
½ red apple
½ cup blueberries
¼ cup pineapple chunks
1 cup frozen shelled edamame
¼ avocado
1 tablespoon extra virgin olive oil
2 tablespoons chia seeds or Fuel Up Protein Seed Mix (see page 130)
½ cup ice cubes (optional)

Star Ingredient: Blueberries

Touted as the world's healthiest food, blueberries are known to have the highest source of antioxidants. They include vitamin C, manganese, vitamin K, and fiber, and are about 85 percent water. Research suggests eating blueberries regularly may improve memory and delay age-related cognitive decline.

MACRO DADDY BLEND

1 cup unsweetened almond or coconut milk
½ banana
1 cup baby spinach or other greens
2 teaspoons hemp seeds
2 teaspoons chia seeds
½ tablespoon almond or cashew butter
2 scoops protein powder
½-inch chunk fresh ginger
1 cup water
½ cup ice cubes (optional)

PLANT-PACKED PERFECTION

1 cup coconut water
½ cup sliced cucumber
¼ cup Fuel Up Protein Seed Mix (see page 130) or hemp seeds
1 cup peas (frozen recommended)
1 cup broccoli (frozen recommended)
1 cup baby spinach
½ cup parsley
¼ cup pineapple chunks
Juice of ½ lemon
2 teaspoons raspberries or dried goji berries
½ cup ice cubes (optional)

EDAMAM-YAY!

1 cup unsweetened nut, seed, or oat milk
1 cup frozen shelled edamame
½ banana
½ cup blueberries
¼ cup pineapple chunks
1 tablespoon cacao powder
1 pinch ground cinnamon
½ cup ice cubes (optional)

FuelUp

GREEK GODDESS

1 cup unsweetened nut, seed, or oat milk
1 cup Greek yogurt
¼ cup Fuel Up Protein Seed Mix (see page 130) or hemp seeds
2 cups baby kale
½ cup blueberries
½ cup pineapple chunks
1 pinch ground cinnamon
½ cup ice cubes (optional)

BERRYLICIOUS

1 cup unsweetened nut, seed, or oat milk
2 cups baby spinach
1 cup cauliflower florets (frozen recommended)
½ cup pineapple chunks
1 tablespoon chia seeds or Fuel Up Protein Seed Mix (see page 130)
1 serving chocolate or vanilla protein powder
½ banana
½ cup ice cubes (optional)

Level 3:
Challenge Your Taste Buds

THE GREEN MACHINE

1 cup unsweetened nut, seed, or oat milk
¼ cup Fuel Up Protein Nut Mix (see page 129) or cashews
1 tablespoon cacao powder
2 cups baby kale
1 cup cauliflower florets (frozen recommended)
½ cup peas (frozen recommended)
½ banana
1 pinch ground cinnamon
½ cup ice cubes (optional)

COLIN'S GREEN SLIME

1 cup water
½ cup chopped tomato
½ cup sliced carrot with tops or baby carrots
½ beet with beet greens
1 cup baby kale
½ cup Swiss chard
1 cup frozen shelled edamame
¼ cup Fuel Up Protein Seed Mix (see page 130) or chia seeds
½ cup ice cubes (optional)

DINO DELIGHT

1 cup coconut water
1 tablespoon spirulina powder
2 cups dinosaur (lacinato) kale
1 cup peas (frozen recommended)
1 cup broccoli florets (frozen recommended)
¼ cup Fuel Up Protein Seed Mix (see page 130)
¼ cup pineapple chunks
1 pinch ground cinnamon
½ cup ice cubes (optional)

GET ROOTED

1 cup water or coconut water
1 cup Swiss chard
½ lemon with pith
1-inch chunk ginger root
½-inch chunk turmeric root
½ apple, cored
1 serving chocolate or vanilla protein powder
½ cup ice cubes (optional)

Directions for Turning Any Smoothie into a Smoothie Bowl

Turn any of our smoothie recipes into a smoothie bowl by adding half an avocado, 1 tablespoon of chia seeds, or ½ cup of frozen, shelled edamame or frozen peas prior to blending. These ingredients will thicken the smoothie so you can pour it into a bowl and add yummy toppings such as shredded coconut, hemp seeds, pumpkin seeds, cacao nibs, or sliced banana to the top. A great treat on a hot day!

Warm Breakfast Bowls

Sometimes on a cold day, a cold smoothie just isn't what you are craving, which is why we are providing you with some warm breakfast options in the form of porridges —warm, cooked grains like quinoa, millet, or oatmeal—with pour-over smoothies for added nutrients and flavor.

THE PERFECT PUMPKIN BREAKFAST BOWL

1 cup almond milk

1 cup cooked oatmeal, cooled

1 cup canned pumpkin

1 tablespoon applesauce

1 pinch ground cinnamon

½ tablespoon maple syrup

Add all the ingredients to a blender and blend until slightly textured.

Heat the blend in a small pot over medium heat.

Pour the blend into a bowl and sprinkle it with hemp seeds, raisins, diced apple, and/or slivered almonds.

SAVORY FARRO BOWL

½ cup cottage cheese or ricotta cheese

1 teaspoon nutritional yeast

1 small scallion, bottom removed

1 pinch dried oregano

1 pinch ground cumin

Salt and pepper to taste

1 cup cooked farro (oatmeal or brown rice)

Blend together all the ingredients except the farro until smooth. Add the blend to a small saucepan and cook it over medium heat.

Add the farro and stir it in. Add salt and pepper to taste.

Add diced tomato, avocado, sautéed root vegetables, microgreens, or even a fried egg to the top to make it extra savory and delicious!

COMFORT FOOD QUINOA BOWL

1 cup cooked quinoa, cooled

¼ cup apple chunks

1 cup almond milk

1 pinch ground cinnamon or your favorite spice mix
(such as pumpkin spice)

½ tablespoon honey or maple syrup

Add all the ingredients to a blender and blend until slightly textured.

Heat the blend in a small pot over medium heat.

Choose your favorite smoothie recipe and make a half-size version of it. Place the porridge in a bowl and pour the smoothie over the top.

Star Ingredient: Quinoa

Did you know that quinoa is really a seed and not a grain? It's a great source of fiber and protein, as well as nutrients such as zinc, magnesium, folate, and iron. It is used in many dishes as a replacement for pasta because it's gluten-free, but we love it as is.

Healthy Meal Enhancements

Our Meal Enhancement recipes include healthy and delicious sauces, marinades, pestos, dressings, and condiments—things you can use to add both nutrients *and* flavor to your meals. You can also use these enhancements to dress up items such as those veggies that you're less fond of. You may find you enjoy them after all!

Sauces and Marinades

The following recipes can be used to boost both the flavor and nutrients of any fish, meat, or vegetable dish.

To use as a **Sauce**: Cook your protein or veggies as desired and then pour the sauce over the top.

To use as a **Marinade**: Prior to cooking, pour the marinade over your protein or veggies and mix well so everything is coated. Then bake, roast, sauté, or air-fry, and enjoy!

Directions for Making Sauces and Marinades

1. Add all ingredients to your blender.
2. Blend until you have a smooth sauce.
3. Enjoy!

All recipes make about 4 servings and can be stored in the refrigerator for up to 1 week.

LGO

Juice of 2 lemons
2 garlic cloves
¼ cup extra virgin olive oil

LEMON GINGER JOY

Juice of 2 lemons
½-inch chunk ginger
¼ cup sesame oil

ENHANCED STIR-FRY SAUCE

1-inch chunk ginger
1 to 2 garlic cloves
2 tablespoons toasted sesame oil
2 tablespoons soy sauce or coconut aminos
3 Thai basil leaves or regular basil leaves

Note: Use with our Chicken Stir-Fry (page 168) or with any stir-fry recipe.

TANGY CILANTRO CITRUS SAUCE

2 ripe avocados, peeled and pitted
½ cup Greek yogurt
¼ cup extra virgin olive oil
2 garlic cloves

Juice of 2 limes
½ cup cilantro
Salt and pepper to taste

HERBALICIOUS ENHANCEMENT SAUCE

½ cup extra virgin olive oil
2 tablespoons red wine or sherry vinegar
2 tablespoons water
½ cup flat leaf parsley
½ cup basil leaves

1 teaspoon dried oregano
3 garlic cloves
½ teaspoon red pepper flakes
Salt and pepper to taste

Note: This also works wonderfully as a poaching liquid for our Simple Poached Salmon on page 156.

CILANTRO LIME TIME

Juice of 2 limes
1 handful cilantro
¼ cup extra virgin olive oil

ITALIAN SCALLION

Juice of 2 lemons
2 scallions, bottoms removed
¼ cup extra virgin olive oil

1 pinch dried oregano
2 garlic cloves

MEXICAN MARINADE

3 tablespoons extra virgin olive oil
3 tablespoons fresh lime juice
3 tablespoons fresh orange juice
1 teaspoon ground cumin

4 garlic cloves
1 jalapeño, seeded
1 pinch salt

Note: We love this as a marinade for fish or chicken and also use it as a
nutrient-packed base for our Tasty Turkey Chili (page 194).

CHIMICHURRI DELIGHT

¼ cup extra virgin olive oil
1 clove garlic
½ cup green olives
¼ cup scallions, bottoms removed
¼ cup basil leaves

¼ cup parsley leaves
1 pinch red pepper flakes
1 teaspoon lemon zest
Juice of 1 lemon
1 pinch salt

Note: This makes a delicious sauce served over lamb or beef. Or add 1 cup of
water or white wine and use it as a poaching liquid.

Pestos

Besides adding to your weekly plant tally, pestos are an easy and delicious way to use up excess herbs and greens. They freeze well too, so feel free to make them in large batches and save leftovers for another time. Use pestos to top meat or fish dishes, or as a dip for chips or crudités.

Directions for Pestos

1. Add all ingredients to your blender.
2. Pulse until well combined but still a bit textured.
3. Enjoy!

All recipes make about 4 servings.

PUTTING THE PEA IN PESTO

⅓ cup extra virgin olive oil
⅓ cup water
1 cup peas, fresh or thawed frozen
2 cups arugula
1 tablespoon fresh thyme leaves (or 1 pinch dried)
1 teaspoon lemon juice
1 pinch salt
1 pinch ground black pepper
½ cup of cashews, walnuts, or pine nuts

AMAZING ARUGULA PESTO

½ cup extra virgin olive oil
2 cups arugula
½ cup walnuts
½ cup shredded Parmesan cheese
2 garlic cloves
½ teaspoon salt

MAGICAL MINT PESTO

½ cup extra virgin olive oil
2 cups fresh mint
½ cup pine nuts or cashews
½ cup shredded Parmesan cheese
2 garlic cloves
½ teaspoon salt

Salad Dressings

In addition to the dressings that follow, the first four recipes under Sauces and Marinades also work as delicious salad dressings: LGO, Lemon Ginger Joy, Cilantro Lime Time, and Italian Scallion.

Directions for Making Salad Dressings

1. Add all ingredients to your blender.
2. Pulse until you achieve a smooth, dressing-like consistency.
3. Enjoy!

All recipes make about 4 servings.

QUICK AND EASY SAVORY TAHINI DRESSING

2 tablespoons extra virgin olive oil
Juice of 2 lemons
2 tablespoons tahini
1 pinch dried thyme

ENHANCED RANCH DRESSING

1 cup Greek yogurt
1 teaspoon lemon zest
1 tablespoon lemon juice
1 small Persian cucumber
4 to 5 baby carrots
2 scallions, bottoms removed
1 pinch celery seed

Note: In addition to being delicious on a green salad, this makes a great dip for veggies or chicken nuggets. You can also stir it into a can of tuna for a healthy and flavorful lunch!

TWISTED GINGER SESAME DRESSING

3 garlic cloves
½ cup ginger chunks
1 carrot (or ½ cup baby carrots)
1 apple (quartered and cored)
¼ white onion
½ cup red wine vinegar
1 tablespoon miso paste
2 tablespoons maple syrup
1 teaspoon sesame oil

APHRODITE DRESSING

½ cup water
1 cup parsley
1 cup basil
1 cup baby spinach
1 cup cilantro
2 to 3 scallions, bottoms removed
⅓ cup cashews, soaked in water for 20 minutes
⅓ cup nutritional yeast
¾ cup Greek yogurt
Juice of ½ lemon
1 to 2 garlic cloves
Salt and pepper to taste
3 tablespoons extra virgin olive oil

Star Ingredient: Garlic

Garlic is the star of the heart-health show! It has the potential to reduce high blood pressure and improve blood flow by helping dilate blood vessels, but it can also bolster immunity and exert anti-inflammatory properties. Garlic is a good source of several nutrients, notably manganese, vitamin B_6, vitamin C, selenium, and fiber.

Condiments

SIMPLE AND CLEAN KETCHUP

Makes about 10 servings

One 3-ounce can tomato paste

2 to 3 tablespoons white vinegar

2 teaspoons maple syrup

½ teaspoon garlic powder

½ teaspoon onion powder

Add all the ingredients to a blender and blend until smooth.

Heat the mixture over low heat for 10 minutes.

Pour the ketchup into a storage container. It will keep for up to 2 weeks in the fridge.

Feel free to explore by adding rosemary, horseradish, or other flavors that sound exciting to you.

DON'T MESS WITH TEXAS BBQ SAUCE

Makes about 8 servings

1½ cups Simple and Clean Ketchup (recipe above)

⅓ cup maple syrup

¼ cup water

3 tablespoons red wine vinegar

2 tablespoons extra virgin olive oil

One 3-ounce can tomato paste

1 tablespoon ground yellow mustard

1 tablespoon chili powder

½ tablespoon ground black pepper

½ teaspoon salt

½ teaspoon onion powder

½ teaspoon garlic powder

¼ teaspoon ground ginger

Add all the ingredients to a blender and blend until smooth.

Store the BBQ sauce in an airtight container in the refrigerator for up to 1 month.

SAVORY BEAST HOT SAUCE

Makes about 10 servings

4 cups mixed hot peppers such as cayenne,
Fresno, jalapeño, or serrano
4 cloves garlic
½ cup chopped onion
1 teaspoon salt
1½ cups apple cider vinegar

Remove the stems from the peppers and chop them. Remove the seeds as desired: The more you remove, the milder the flavor will be. The more you leave in, the hotter!

Add the garlic and onion to a blender and pulse a few times until the mixture is blended but still a bit chunky.

Add the peppers, the garlic and onion blend, and 1 cup of water to a pot and simmer over low heat until the peppers are soft, about 20 minutes.

Set the sauce aside for about 15 minutes to cool.

Add the cooled sauce to the blender with 1 cup of the vinegar and blend until smooth. Add more salt and vinegar until the desired taste is achieved. Strain out the seeds with a sieve.

Pour the hot sauce into an airtight container and keep it refrigerated for up to 1 month.

CRANBERRY RELISH

Makes about 6 servings

½ cup fresh cranberries
½ cup maple syrup
¼ cup prepared horseradish
1 tablespoon lemon juice

Add all the ingredients to the blender and pulse until blended but still textured.

Cover and chill for 12 hours or overnight.

Broths, Soups, and Stews

Soups and stews are an easy way to add plants to your meals, but we take that idea to the next level with our Enhanced Broths. Instead of using basic, store-bought broths like chicken or beef as a base for our soups, we soup them up (pun intended!) by blending them with veggies and herbs to really pack in the nutrients. We use those Enhanced Broths in our soup and stew recipes, but they are also delicious on their own. Sip them as a hydrating snack, as a comfort food when you're not feeling well, as a coffee replacement, or even paired with a salad for a light lunch.

Enhanced Broths

Directions for Making Enhanced Broths

1. Add all ingredients to your blender.

2. Blend until smooth, about 1 minute.

3. Enjoy!

All recipes make about 4 servings.

VEGGIE STRONG BROTH BLEND

2 yellow squash
2 cups baby spinach
1 cup carrot
1 clove garlic
3 cups vegetable broth
1 pinch dried oregano
1 pinch celery seed
1 pinch onion powder
1 pinch garlic powder

FANTASTIC FISH BROTH BLEND

2 yellow squash
2 cups baby spinach
1 stalk celery
1 clove garlic
1 bay leaf
1 pinch Old Bay seasoning (optional)
3 cups fish stock or broth

SAVORY BEEF BROTH BLEND

3 cups beef broth
2 tablespoons tomato paste
2 garlic cloves
1 cup red wine
2 sprigs parsley
2 sprigs thyme

"TRASH CAN" POACHING BROTH

Leftover carrot tops
Leftover broccoli stems
Leftover beet greens
1 garlic clove
1 teaspoon lemon zest
2 sprigs fresh thyme or any other fresh herb
3 cups chicken, beef, or veggie broth
1 cup chardonnay (optional)
Salt and pepper to taste

Note: This recipe is perfect for our Simple Poached Salmon recipe on page 156.

Hearty Soups and Stews

TASTY TURKEY CHILI

Makes about 4 servings

1 tablespoon extra virgin olive oil
½ cup diced onion
1 pound ground turkey
½ cup Mexican Marinade (page 185)
One 14-ounce can kidney beans, drained and rinsed
One 14-ounce can diced tomato
1 tablespoon Worcestershire sauce
1 capful liquid smoke (optional)
Salt and pepper to taste

Heat the olive oil in a pot over medium heat and lightly brown the onions. Add the turkey and marinade and cook for about 8 minutes.

Add all the remaining ingredients. Cover and let the mixture simmer, stirring occasionally, for about 20 minutes.

Enjoy with sliced avocado and chopped cilantro on top.

Star Ingredient: Mushrooms

Mushrooms are the star of the immunity show! We are talking about edible mushrooms used for food, and not psychedelic ones, of course. The glucans found in mushrooms are responsible for their immune-regulating, anti-tumor/cancer, and general health-promoting effects. Glucans are best expressed when cooked, so it's time to learn new recipes for cooking delicious mushrooms! See the cooking section at the end of our 7-Day Beast Blending Lifestyle plan for some more options.

FANTASTICALLY FRESH FISH CHOWDER

Makes about 4 servings

1 cup diced yellow onion

1 cup diced bell pepper

1 cup chopped carrot

1 cup chopped celery

1 tablespoon extra virgin olive oil

1 pound white fish such as cod, sea bass, or flounder, chopped into ½-inch chunks

2 cups Fantastic Fish Broth Blend (page 193)

1 pinch celery seed

¼ cup fresh minced herbs such as thyme, sage, and rosemary

1 teaspoon Old Bay spice (optional)

Brown all the vegetables in the olive oil in a good-sized pot.

Add the fish chunks and brown them a little on each side.

Add the broth and remaining spices and stir.

Cook the chowder over medium heat for about 10 minutes. Then stir, reduce the heat to low, cover, and simmer for about 40 minutes, stirring every 10 minutes.

Serve the chowder in a bowl with a drizzle of olive oil and salt and pepper to taste.

Feel free to add canned clams (drained and rinsed) or replace the fish with clams. Enjoy!

Note: To make this dish more like a cioppino, add a can of diced tomato.

BEAUTIFUL BEEF BOURGUIGNON

Makes about 4 servings

1 cup diced yellow onion
2 cups sliced mushrooms
1 cup diced carrots
1 cup diced celery
1 tablespoon extra virgin olive oil
2 cups cubed beef (top sirloin or London broil are great choices)
2 cups Savory Beef Broth Blend (page 193)
Salt and pepper to taste

Brown the onion, mushroom, carrots, and celery in the olive oil in a good-sized pot.

Add the beef cubes and brown them on both sides.

Add the broth and cook over medium heat for about 10 minutes.

Give everything a stir and turn the heat down to low. Cover and simmer the stew for about 2 hours, stirring occasionally.

Check the meat to make sure it's done to your liking, and serve the stew over brown rice.

PROTEIN PACKED BUTTERNUT SQUASH SOUP

Makes about 4 servings

1 butternut squash (about 2 pounds)
1 tablespoon extra virgin olive oil
2 cloves garlic
1 diced yellow onion
3 medium sprigs rosemary
2 sprigs fresh oregano or 2 pinches dried oregano
One 14-ounce can white beans, drained and rinsed
3 cups Veggie Strong Broth Blend (page 192), plus more as needed
1 cup almond milk
Salt and pepper to taste

Preheat the oven to 425°F.

Cut the squash in half the long way and scoop out the seeds.

Grease the baking sheet with olive oil and place the squash halves on it flat side down. Place the garlic, onion, rosemary, and oregano leaves next to the squash on the baking sheet and place the baking sheet in the oven.

After 30 minutes, check on the roasted herbs. Remove them and set them aside if they seem nice and roasted.

Stick a fork into the squash. If the fork goes in easily, it's done. If not, give it another 10 minutes and try the fork again. Keep cooking until the squash is tender enough for the fork to go in effortlessly.

Set the squash aside to cool, remove the peel, and cut it into chunks and add it to the blender.

Add the roasted onion, garlic, and herbs along with the beans and veggie broth. Split the soup into two portions if needed to fit into your blender. (It will all come together in the pot!)

Blend until smooth and then pour the soup into a saucepan to heat. Stir in the almond milk while it's heating.

Enjoy with a drizzle of olive oil, diced avocado, and a sprinkle of your favorite microgreens. Add salt and pepper to taste.

Satiating Snacks

Snacking gets a bad rap, probably because people often reach for ultraprocessed foods when they're hungry between meals. But with just a little forethought, snacks can absolutely be part of a healthy eating pattern. Try our plant-centric dips, salsas, and spreads, which can be paired with fresh-cut veggies, our Herbed Seed Crackers (page 224), or one of the bread recipes you will find later in this chapter. Or try our Salad Shooters—three-gulp, veggie-packed smoothies that serve as a hydrating pick-me-up, a pre-dinner amuse-bouche, or a healthy pre-gaming strategy before an indulgent evening.

Spreads, Salsas, and Dips

PATRICIA'S SIMPLE PEA SPREAD

Makes about 4 servings

1 cup frozen peas

1 tablespoon water

1 pinch each salt and pepper

Add all the ingredients to a small blender and blend until smooth.

HOORAY FOR HUMMUS

Makes about 4 servings

One 14-ounce can chickpeas, drained and rinsed

3 level tablespoons tahini

Juice of 2 lemons

2 teaspoons lemon zest

½ teaspoon garlic powder or 2

garlic cloves

2 sprigs fresh herbs such as rosemary, thyme, or oregano (optional)

1 pinch salt

1 tablespoon extra virgin olive oil

Add all the ingredients except the olive oil to a blender and blend until smooth.

Pour the hummus into a bowl and drizzle it with olive oil.

TRI-COLOR PEPPER HUMMUS

Makes about 4 servings

One 14-ounce can chickpeas, drained and rinsed
2 tablespoons tahini
¼ cup red pepper chunks
¼ cup yellow pepper chunks
¼ cup orange pepper chunks
1 garlic clove
1 teaspoon lemon zest
Juice of 1 lemon
Salt to taste

Add all the ingredients to a blender and blend to a smooth and creamy consistency.

Drizzle with extra virgin olive oil and sprinkle with fresh herbs if you like.

DREAMY TZATZIKI

Makes about 4 servings

2 cups Greek yogurt
1 tablespoon lemon juice
1 tablespoon tahini
1 garlic clove
3 mint leaves
5 sprigs dill
4 scallions, bottoms removed
1 small cucumber, seeded
1 pinch salt
1 pinch ground black pepper

Add all the ingredients to a blender and pulse until well combined but still a little textured.

Makes a great veggie dip or topper in a chicken wrap.

DID SOMEONE SAY SALSA?

Makes about 4 servings

2 cups chopped fresh tomatoes (Roma tomatoes are perfect)
1 cup cilantro
2 scallions, bottoms removed
1 jalapeño (less or more depending on desired heat)
1 garlic clove
1 splash apple cider vinegar (optional)

Add all the ingredients to a blender and pulse until they are combined but still a bit chunky.

MIGHTY MANGO SALSA

Makes about 4 servings

¼ cup extra virgin olive oil
½ cup orange juice
1 tablespoon orange zest
2 tablespoons lime zest
2 teaspoons honey
2 teaspoons soy sauce
1 cup fresh cilantro
2 ripe mangos, diced
2 ripe avocados, diced

Add all the ingredients except the mangos and avocados to a blender and blend until smooth.

Place the diced mangos and avocados in a bowl and pour the blended ingredients on top. Stir together and chill for at least 1 hour before serving.

Makes a great accompaniment to fish or chicken dishes.

VERY VEGAN QUESO

Makes about 4 servings

¾ cup rolled oats
¼ cup Did Someone Say Salsa? (page 200)
2 tablespoons nutritional yeast
2 tablespoons diced roasted red pepper
2 tablespoons apple cider vinegar
½ teaspoon ground cumin
½ teaspoon chili powder
½ teaspoon onion powder
1 pinch paprika
1 teaspoon salt

Place the oats in a blender, add 1 cup of water, and let the mixture sit for 20 minutes.

Add the remaining ingredients and blend until smooth.

Pour the queso into a pot and heat it over medium heat, stirring often.

Serve hot with Oat Naan (page 225).

BEYOND BEAN DIP

Makes about 4 servings

One 14-ounce can black or pinto beans, drained and rinsed
½ cup Greek yogurt
1 tablespoon nutritional yeast
1 teaspoon ground cumin
1 pinch red pepper flakes
10 sprigs cilantro
1 teaspoon Worcestershire sauce
1 capful liquid smoke (optional)

Add all the ingredients to the blender and pulse until well combined but still a little textured.

Makes a great side for chicken dishes.

Salad Shooters

Directions for Making Salad Shooters

1. Add all the ingredients to your blender.

2. Blend until smooth, about 1 minute.

3. Enjoy!

All recipes make about 2 servings.

POPEYE'S PASSION

1 tablespoon extra virgin olive oil
1 tablespoon apple cider vinegar
1 cup water
1 cup baby spinach
1 celery stalk
1 small cucumber or ½ larger one
Juice of ½ lemon
5 sprigs parsley
1 pinch salt

FEEL THE BEET

1 tablespoon extra virgin olive oil
1 cup coconut water
¼ cup raw beet chunks
1 cup baby carrots or carrot chunks
1 cup arugula or any other greens
1 cup baby spinach or any other greens
1 celery stalk
1 small cucumber
1 tablespoon chia seeds

Star Ingredient: Beets

Beets are a great source of nitrates, which are known to dilate blood vessels. This is a good thing because it can lower blood pressure, improve cognition, and maybe even help with erectile dysfunction! Drinking beet juice before exercise may also help with endurance. We love them in a smoothie because they add sweetness, but they're also great cut up in a salad. Be careful: they can stain your clothing!

PARSLEY PERFECT

1 tablespoon extra virgin olive oil
1 cup water
1 cup fresh parsley
1 small cucumber
1 cup baby spinach
Juice of 1 lemon
1 tablespoon chia seed or any other seeds

THE RED HEAD

1 tablespoon extra virgin olive oil
1 cup water
1 cup baby carrots or carrot chunks
¼ orange bell pepper, seeded
½ cup cooked sweet potato, cooled and peeled
1 tablespoon hemp seeds
1 pinch pumpkin spice (optional)

GAZPACH-WHOA

1 tablespoon extra virgin olive oil
1 tablespoon red wine vinegar or sherry vinegar
1 cup water
1 small cucumber or ½ larger cucumber
¼ bell pepper, seeded
1 clove garlic
Small wedge red onion
1 cup cilantro
1 cup baby spinach or any other greens
1 pinch salt

Sweets and Treats

As with snacks, sweets and treats *can* be part of a healthy eating pattern. Our intention here is to offer you versions that are just a little health*ier* than what you would typically find at the grocery store. They feature natural ingredients and largely stay away from UPFs. They are also plant strong and nutrient dense, often with added fiber and protein to fill you up a little faster. But don't be fooled, however: they will still satisfy your sweet tooth!

No-Cook Puddings and Dessert Smoothies

MATCHA PUDDING

Makes about 2 servings

1 cup almond milk
2 teaspoons matcha green tea powder
¼ cup chia seeds
½ cup raw cashews
2 medjool dates, pitted

Add all the ingredients to a blender and blend until smooth.

Chill the pudding in the refrigerator for at least 1 hour.

Serve with a sprinkle of chia seeds and fresh berries.

CHICKA CHICKA BOOM BOOM CHOCOLATE PUDDING

Makes about 4 servings

1 can chickpeas, drained
1½ cups almond milk
1 cup chocolate chips
4 medjool dates, pitted
1 teaspoon vanilla extract
1 teaspoon coconut oil
1 pinch salt

Add all the ingredients to a blender and blend until smooth.

Chill in the refrigerator for 2 hours.

Serve with a sprinkle of fresh berries and a mint sprig on top.

VEGAN NUTELLA DESSERT SMOOTHIE

Makes about 4 servings

2 frozen bananas
2 cups almond milk
2 tablespoons nut butter
1 serving chocolate protein powder

Add all the ingredients to a blender and blend until smooth.

Serve with a sprinkle of fresh berries, crushed hazelnuts, and a mint sprig on top.

"NICE" CREAM SMOOTHIE

Makes about 2 servings

2 frozen bananas
1 handful chocolate chips (optional)
2 to 3 mint leaves (optional)
1 splash almond milk

Add all the ingredients to a blender and blend until smooth.

COLIN'S DATE NIGHT SMOOTHIE

Makes about 1 serving

6 medjool dates, pitted
½ frozen banana
1 pinch ground cinnamon
1 splash nut milk

Add all the ingredients to a blender and blend until smooth.

Frozen Desserts

REFRIGERATOR CLEANUP FRUIT POPS

Makes about 4 servings

1 cup any fresh fruit from the fridge (such as cored apple chunks, berries, grapes, or cored pear chunks)

1 banana or avocado

1 cup coconut water

Add all the ingredients to a blender and blend until smooth.

Pour into popsicle molds and freeze for at least 4 hours.

BLACKBERRY FREEZER POPS

Makes about 4 servings

2 cups frozen blackberries

¼ cup water

3 tablespoon maple syrup

1 teaspoon lemon juice

1 spring mint (optional)

Add all the ingredients to a blender and blend until smooth.

Pour into popsicle molds and freeze for at least 4 hours.

Star Ingredient: Allulose

While it's generally a good idea to limit sweeteners—especially table sugar—we obviously don't expect you to give up sweets entirely. Otherwise, we wouldn't have a whole category of recipes called Sweets and Treats! Allulose is our new favorite sweetener. It is a naturally occurring monosaccharide (simple sugar). Research suggests that not only does it *not* affect your blood sugar, but it may actually improve blood sugar and insulin response. It tastes slightly less sweet than sucrose (aka table sugar) and can be used as a 1:1 substitute.

COTTAGE CHEESE ICE CREAM

Makes about 4 servings

2 cups cottage cheese
2 tablespoons honey or maple syrup

Add the cottage cheese and honey to the blender and blend until smooth.

Choose from any of the following optional add-in ingredients and blend until you achieve the desired texture: peanut butter, chocolate chips, berries, mint, vanilla bean, coffee beans.

Pour the ice cream mixture into a freezer-friendly container and freeze for at least 4 hours.

Remove the ice cream from the freezer and let it sit for 10 minutes before serving.

LOW-GLYCEMIC PUMPKIN ICE CREAM

Makes about 4 servings

One 15-ounce can pumpkin purée
2 tablespoons allulose or monk fruit sweetener
1 teaspoon ground ginger
1 teaspoon ground cinnamon
1 teaspoon vanilla extract
1 pinch ground cloves

Add all the ingredients to a blender and blend until smooth.

Spoon the ice cream mixture into a freezer-friendly container and freeze for at least 4 hours.

Remove the ice cream from the freezer and let it sit for 10 minutes before serving. Top it with coconut whipped cream or a sprinkle of granola.

Baked Treats

BANANA OAT MINI MUFFINS

Makes about 10 muffins

½ cup almond milk
1 egg
1 teaspoon vanilla extract
1 tablespoon maple syrup
½ banana
1 cup oatmeal
½ cup dark chocolate chips (optional)

Preheat the oven to 425°F.

Add the almond milk, egg, vanilla, maple syrup, and banana to a blender and blend until smooth.

Add the oatmeal to the ingredients in the blender. Stir them into the mixture with a spoon and set it aside for a few minutes for the oats to soak up the moisture a bit.

Pour the mixture into greased mini muffin cups. Add 4 chocolate chips to each, if desired.

Bake for 12 minutes or until the tops are golden brown.

Serve the muffins warm or refrigerate them for up to 5 days.

LOVELY LENTIL BROWNIE BITES

Makes about 12 bites

2 eggs
½ cup almond milk
6 pitted medjool dates
1 cup cooked lentils
1 cup cacao powder
¼ cup maple syrup
1 teaspoon vanilla extract
½ cup chopped walnuts (optional)
1 teaspoon coarse salt

Preheat the oven to 425°F.

Add all the ingredients except the walnuts and salt to a blender and blend until smooth.

Pour the contents into greased mini muffin tins. Sprinkle salt and walnuts (if desired) on top of each.

Bake for about 20 minutes or until a toothpick inserted comes out clean.

Beverages

Because staying hydrated may be the single most important thing you can do to improve your health, we offer a whole variety of ways to do this, including our Enhanced Water Infusions, Hydration Blends, Pick-Me-Ups, and Mocktails. And these can work better than water alone, because they make it more pleasurable to hydrate and because we pair liquids with plants that contain fiber, electrolytes, and other nutrients that help you absorb water better. A quick word about the mocktails included in this section: recent research suggests that no amount of alcohol is safe for your health, which is why we offer these delicious alternatives. Of course, if you want to booze them up by adding a shot of vodka, rum, or another liquor, you can do that and they will still be healthier than your average mixer!

Enhanced Water Infusions

Directions for Making Enhanced Water Infusions

1. Add all ingredients to your blender.

2. Pulse a few times until the ingredients are combined but still chunky.

3. Spoon the pulsed ingredients into an infuser, tea ball, or fillable tea bag; submerge it in water and let steep for a few minutes.

4. Chill the water, drink it at room temperature, or add ice to enjoy.

All recipes make about 1 serving.

CUCUMBER MINT

½ small cucumber
1 sprig fresh mint

BASIL BERRY

½ cup strawberries
2 sprigs fresh basil leaves

LEMON CHERRY

¼ lemon wedge
¼ cup pitted cherries

SALTED MANGO

½ cup mango chunks
1 pinch salt

MELON MADNESS

¼ cup watermelon chunks
¼ cup cantaloupe chunks
¼ lemon wedge
1 pinch salt

MUDDLED LAVENDER, BLUEBERRY, AND CHIA

2 sprigs lavender
¼ cup blueberries
½ tablespoon chia seed

LEMON GINGER ELIXIR

¼ lemon wedge
½-inch piece ginger

Hydration Blends

These Hydration Blends are perfect for sipping during and after workouts. They are so tasty, in fact, that they can motivate you to get moving! They are also on the larger side to serve as a real thirst quencher.

ELECTROLYTE DELIGHT

Makes about 2 servings

2 cups coconut water
2 cups water
1 tablespoon maple syrup
Juice of 1 lemon
Juice of 2 oranges
4 pinches salt

Add all the ingredients to a blender and pulse a few times until well blended.

CITRUS ELECTROLYTE REFRESHER

Makes about 2 servings

2½ cups cold water
½ cup lemon juice
½ cup lime juice
½ cup orange juice
½ teaspoon salt
2 tablespoons honey or maple syrup

Add all the ingredients to a blender and blend until smooth.

Chill or pour over ice.

COCONUT CRANBERRY POST-WORKOUT HYDRATOR

Makes about 2 servings

2 cups cold water
1 cup unsweetened cranberry juice
1 cup coconut water
1 pinch salt

Add all the ingredients to a blender and blend until smooth.

Chill or pour over ice.

Pick-Me-Ups and Mocktails

BANANA DATE LATTE

Makes 1 serving

2 medjool dates, pitted
1 banana
1 to 2 shots espresso
1 cup nut milk
1 cup ice

Add all the ingredients to a blender and blend until smooth.

Note: You can add more ice if you want a slushier consistency.

MOCHA BLISS BLEND

Makes about 1 serving

1 cup coffee, cooled
1 cup coconut milk
1 banana
1 serving chocolate protein powder
½ cup ice

Add all the ingredients to a blender and blend until smooth.

Note: You can add more ice if you want a slushier consistency.

GREEN TEA ENERGIZING ELIXIR

Makes about 1 serving

2 cups green tea, cooled
½ red apple, cored
Juice of 1 lemon
2 teaspoons honey
1 cup ice

Add all the ingredients except the ice to a blender and blend until smooth.

Pour over ice and garnish with a lavender sprig and/or cinnamon stick, if desired.

Star Ingredient: Green Tea

Touted as the healthiest beverage, green tea contains a polyphenol called catechins, the most abundant of which is epigallocatechin gallate, or EGCG. These plant compounds are potent antioxidants that can help with cognitive function and blood sugar management. There is even research being done on their association with lowered risk of some cancers.

LEMON GINGER LIGHTHOUSE

Makes about 2 servings

1 cup lemon ginger tea, cooled
1 cup coconut water
Juice of 1 lemon
¼ cup blueberries
¼ cup blackberries
2 sprigs fresh mint

Add all the ingredients except the mint and ice to the blender and blend until slightly chunky.

Pour into two glasses over ice.

Garnish with the sprig of mint in each glass. (Slap the mint between your hands first to release the essential oils and flavor.)

CHAMOMILE AND CHILL SHRUB

Makes about 2 servings

1 cup chilled chamomile tea
½ cup tart cherry juice
2 tablespoons orange juice
1 tablespoon apple cider vinegar
½ cup ice
1 cup sparkling water

Add all the ingredients except the sparkling water to a blender.

Pour into two glasses. Add sparkling water to the top of each and stir gently.

Garnish with a cherry and a cinnamon stick.

Note: A shrub, also called drinking vinegar, is a drink made with vinegar and fruit. Shrubs are enjoyed throughout the world and were even popular in colonial America.

PIÑA MOCKLADA

Makes about 1 serving

½ cup pineapple juice
½ cup pineapple chunks
½ cup cream of coconut
1 cup ice

Add all the ingredients to a blender and blend until smooth and creamy.

Garnish with a cherry, mint, and a chunk of pineapple.

Note: Add a shot of rum if you're feeling frisky or freeze into pops!

HIBISCUS CHILL TIME MULE

Makes about 2 servings

Juice of 1 lime
½ cup frozen pineapple chunks
½ cup hibiscus tea
One 6-ounce can ginger beer
1 pinch ginger zest (optional)
1 sprig rosemary
1 cup ice

Add the lime, pineapple, and tea to a blender and blend until smooth.

Split into two glasses, add ice to each, and top with ginger beer. Stir gently with a spoon.

Add a pinch of ginger zest and a sprig of rosemary.

ROSEMARY CLARITY FROZEN MOCKARITA

Makes about 2 servings

Juice of ½ lime
Juice of ½ lemon
3 cups rosemary tea (steep 1 cup rosemary in hot water and let cool)
6 to 8 drops stevia or your favorite sweetener
1 cup ice
1 pinch salt

Add all the ingredients to a blender and blend until smooth. Add more ice if you want a more slushy consistency.

Salt the rim of your glass (optional).

VIRGIN WATERMELON DAIQUIRI

Makes about 2 servings

2 cups watermelon chunks
Juice of 2 limes
½ cup orange juice
1 cup ice

Add all the ingredients to a blender and blend until smooth and creamy.

Add more ice if you want a slushier consistency.

Garnish with a cherry, a sprig of mint, and a chunk of pineapple.

IMMUNE-BOOSTING ELDERBERRY SANGRIA

Makes about 4 servings

1 lime, quartered
¼ cup blueberries
¼ cup blackberries
¼ cup pineapple chunks
2 tablespoons elderberry syrup
1 tablespoon honey
24 ounces seltzer water, plain or flavored
2 cups ice

Add all the ingredients except seltzer water and ice to a blender and pulse until blended but still textured.

Add the blended ingredients to a pitcher. Add the seltzer water.

Stir things up a bit. Add the ice.

Note: If you want this to be a more traditional sangria, substitute half the seltzer for prosecco or wine.

Star Ingredient: Elderberry

Elderberries are filled with antioxidants and vitamins such as calcium, iron, magnesium, vitamin C, potassium, and vitamin A. These nutrients support your immune system and may help you combat symptoms of the common cold or flu. Elderberries must be prepared as a syrup or jam and should not be eaten raw.

Unexpected Blender Recipes

A blender is a much more versatile tool than many people realize. In these recipes, we use it to whip up unexpected items like natural, additive-free crackers, breads, and sandwich wraps. We also use it to quickly blend together lunch spreads such as egg salad and chicken salad to fill those sandwiches—which make great meal options for our 7-Day Beast Blending Lifestyle Plan.

Wraps, Crackers, and Breads

SPINACH WRAPS

Makes about 2

2 handfuls baby spinach
1 egg
1 cup almond flour

Preheat the oven to 300°F.

Blend all the ingredients together until smooth.

Pour the mixture onto a wax paper–lined baking sheet in a thin layer and bake for 20 minutes.

Use the wrap as a sandwich wrap or add ingredients like hummus, chicken, and cucumber, then roll it up and cut it into sushi-style bites.

RED LENTIL WRAPS

Makes about 8

¾ cup dry red lentils
1½ cups broth (chicken, vegetable, or Enhanced Broths on page 192)
1 tablespoon extra virgin olive oil

Rinse the lentils and place them in a blender. Add the broth and let the lentils soak for 2 hours.

Blend until smooth.

Heat the olive oil in a skillet over medium heat. Pour in about ⅛ of the batter and spread it with a spoon to cover the bottom of the pan. Cook for about 4 minutes on each side.

Repeat until you've used up all the batter, pulsing the batter in the blender a few times before you cook each wrap so they all turn out the same.

Serve right away or put wax paper in between the wraps and store in an airtight container for up to 1 week in the refrigerator.

Note: This recipe is somewhat labor-intensive, but it's well worth the effort and much more affordable than store-bought gluten-free wraps. You can also make this recipe more like crepes by using water with a pinch of salt in place of the broth. Add cinnamon and fill with berries, bananas, and other yummy stuff!

HERBED SEED CRACKERS

Makes about 8 servings

½ cup whole flax seeds
½ cup sunflower seeds
½ cup pumpkin seeds
½ cup chia seeds
½ cup hemp seeds
¼ cup (or more) water
½ teaspoon each of your favorite seasoning such as dried rosemary, onion powder, garlic powder, or celery seed

Preheat the oven to 300°F.

Add the flax seeds to a blender and blend them into a fine powder. This is the "glue" for your crackers, so make sure to grind fresh flax seeds first.

Add the remaining seeds to the blender. Add enough water to the vessel to combine all the seeds together and stir with a spoon. It should feel like a thick paste.

Add your herbs and let the mixture sit for 10 minutes.

Spread the mixture onto a wax paper–lined cookie sheet and press it as thin as you can. Try to shape it into a square or rectangle and flatten it with a lightly greased spatula (it's kind of fun!).

Bake the crackers for about an hour, checking on them after 30 minutes. If you want to cut them into squares, do it now with a pizza cutter.

After an hour, remove the crackers and let them cool. If you didn't already cut them, break them into rustic-looking chunks.

Enjoy these crackers with hummus or one of our Lunch Spreads.

Star Ingredient: Pumpkin Seeds

Pumpkin seeds are a great source of fiber and a tasty way to support your gut health and digestion. They can make you feel fuller for longer periods of time and possibly even promote weight loss. We love eating them roasted, right out of the oven, shell and all, as a snack.

OAT NAAN

Makes about 4

1 cup oats
2 cups water
1 pinch onion powder
1 pinch garlic powder
1 pinch dried oregano or your favorite herb

Add all the ingredients to the blender and let them sit for 15 minutes.

Blend until smooth.

Pour the mixture in batches into a heated, oiled sauté pan and cook the naan like pancakes for about 4 minutes on each side. Flatten and thin them out with a spatula or just flip them for more of a naan shape.

This naan is great with hummus or any dip; it's like pita bread.

Note: You can make a sweet version instead by adding 1 teaspoon of vanilla extract and a pinch of cinnamon instead of the savory seasonings. Top with berries.

COTTAGE CHEESE BREAD

Makes about 6 servings

1 cup water
1 cup powdered egg whites
1 cup cultured cottage cheese
1 pinch dried oregano

Preheat the oven to 425°F.

Add all the ingredients to a blender and pulse a few times until blended together.

Pour the batter into a lightly greased, medium loaf pan.

Sprinkle the oregano on top and bake for 35 minutes.

This bread is best served warm and right out of the oven.

Lunch Spreads

Directions for Making Lunch Spreads

1. Add all ingredients to your blender.
2. Pulse until combined but still a bit chunky
3. Enjoy!

All recipes make about 3 servings.

SUPER STEAK SALAD PÂTÉ

1½ cup cooked leftover steak, chopped
1 celery stalk
1 scallion, bottom removed
¼ cup Greek yogurt (add another tablespoon if you like it thinner)
2 sprigs oregano or other fresh herbs
1 tablespoon Superb Steak Sauce (page 60)
Salt and pepper to taste

BLENDER CHICKEN SALAD SPREAD

1 cup cooked chicken, chopped
1 celery stalk
1 scallion, bottom removed
¼ cup plain Greek yogurt (add another tablespoon if you like it thinner)
2 sprigs dill or other fresh herbs
1 pinch celery seed
Salt and pepper to taste

Note: Mix in dried cranberries or halved grapes for added flavor and texture.

EGG-CELLENT EGG SALAD SPREAD

3 hard-boiled eggs, halved
1 celery stalk
1 scallion, bottom removed
¼ cup Greek yogurt (add another tablespoon if you like it thinner)
2 sprigs dill or other fresh herbs
1 tablespoon coarse ground mustard
Salt and pepper to taste

Continue Fueling Up for Years to Come

When we set out to write a book about using your blender to help you "cheat" your way to good health, we had some specific kinds of people in mind. We thought about those who have never picked up a book about healthy eating before. We considered all the yo-yo dieters we have known, who have tried so many different eating plans over the years, only to find that none of them were sustainable. We wanted to provide simple, actionable advice for people who struggle to eat well, which, in our experience, encompasses a lot of people from all walks of life.

Along the way, we discovered that even people who consider themselves relatively healthy are often looking for and even relieved to find advice like this. When we had participants test our 7-Day Beast Blending Lifestyle program, for example, one of the most common reactions we heard was that people felt like this way of eating was something that could continue to work for them over the long term. Unlike so much of what's out there, it wasn't too restrictive, too complicated, too time-consuming, or too expensive to actually last.

FuelUp

We think that people are longing for this kind of guidance because health advice has gotten so complicated and so full of mixed messages that many people don't even know how to eat anymore. And they are tired of being made to feel like they're failing or even ashamed every time they sit down to a meal. That's why what we have really offered you here is a return to basics, because we believe it's the first step to healing.

Our aim has been to do two basic things: help make healthy eating easier for you and help you feel good about what you eat—because both things are important and both are doable! No matter what your eating habits are like, no matter what health conditions you deal with, no matter how many times you have tried to make changes in the past, we hope this book has shown you that it's possible—not to be a perfect eater, because that's an unrealistic goal—and what does "perfect" mean in this context anyway?—but to make a few new, not-too-difficult choices that you will enjoy, that will positively impact your health, and that can make you feel fully fueled and ready to live your life to the fullest. Small changes, reinforced over time, can have real and lasting impact.

And if you don't make the "healthiest" choice every single time, we hope you will remember that there's nothing wrong with that! All of us eat for all sorts of reasons—for comfort, for pleasure, to celebrate, to be reminded of where we come from, to try something new—and that is exactly how it should be. For us, there are no such things as "cheat" foods that you should feel bad about. There are only cheating tactics that can make it that much easier to sneak in more nutrient-rich options and uplevel the quality of foods you use to fuel yourself. And there is no "falling off the wagon" of your diet either. You can use the advice, tips, and recipes in this book regularly, or you can return to them any time you feel like your habits could use a reset. As with all things in life, you should do what works best for you and your body.

We also want you to consider the idea that it's never too late to start "cheating" in this way. Ted, Dr. Dana's longest-running patient and someone she has been treating since she was just out of medical residency, has always been the consummate yo-yo dieter. She watched over the years as he tried various low-carb diets, from Atkins to keto, time and time again. He would lose weight while he was on them, then get off them and binge because the diets were so restrictive. He would end up gaining back the pounds and sometimes more in the process. He was so focused on impossible-to-sustain diets that he never learned the basics of healthy eating. Dr. Dana said to him more than once: "We really need to get you off the diets and just teach you how to eat!"

Finally, only recently, something clicked. Ted has settled into an uncomplicated, plant-positive, overall healthy eating pattern that includes indulgences but none of the shame that used to go along with them. He starts every morning with a Blend with Benefits packed full of plants. He started reading labels. He plays tennis at least four times a week. He told Dr. Dana: "I feel like I missed the boat for twenty years." But now things are different. It's a testament to what simple, sustainable changes—or "cheats"—can do. Now in his late 60s, Ted said to her, "I've never felt better in my life!"

Index

Note: Recipe titles ending with an asterisk (*) indicate smoothie recipes.

INDEX

U

V

Acknowledgments

Dr. Dana

My message of gratitude: I would like to thank my literary agent, Linda Loewenthal, and my new publishing family at Hay House, especially our editor, Melody Guy, and my dear friend Patty Gift, who is truly a gift for me. Christa Bourg, it was my privilege and joy to work with you on the writing of this book. Colin, you and your team at Beast Health are a dream partnership.

I would also like to thank Jay Tejada and Leyla Muedin for putting up with me. Denise Lucero, my office manager, who has been with me for 15 years: I am so proud of you and so grateful you accepted. My patients, whom I have the honor of guiding: you make it all worth it.

Shout-outs to Amy Summers of Pitch Publicity; Shanel Sinclair, social media maven; business consultant Jenna Richardson; and dear friend and PR extraordinaire Beth Grossman. I owe you all a debt of gratitude.

A special thanks to:

My best friends and chosen family, Patricia (and Clementine) Richardson, Trish Mahoney, Dr. Leslie Dick, Devon Nola, Susan Lazarus—thank you all for listening.

My sibs, Lisa Cohen and Jeff Cohen, their kids, and my extended family.

My dear cousin and friend Randi Henry.

Ted Ferrara, who has become a dear friend.

My pup, Frida, you bring me so much joy.

My husband, Henry Caplan, I am so in love with you.

Colin

Thanks to my three Dream Teams:

My amazing wife, Caron, and my daughters, Jessica and Rachel, who have encouraged and supported me in turning my personal passion for nutrition and whole foods into a fruitful career.

Our Beast Health team, whose hard work and dedication has helped turn personal blending into a health movement that can't be stopped.

To Dana, who is a dream co-author, friend, and a true nutrition powerhouse. And, to Christa's outstanding ability to put pen to paper and translate our passion for "Fueling Up." Together we have "blended" our life experiences and knowledge to create this book.

About the Authors

Dr. Dana Cohen has been practicing integrative medicine for over 25 years. Currently in private practice in Manhattan, she is a nationally renowned internal and integrative medicine specialist whose multidisciplinary approach has helped successfully treat thousands of patients. Cohen trained under the late Dr. Robert Atkins, author of the iconic *Dr. Atkins' New Diet Revolution*, and Dr. Ronald L. Hoffman, a pioneer of integrative medicine and founder of the Hoffman Center in New York.

Cohen earned her medical degree from St. George's University School of Medicine and was board-certified by the American Board of Internal Medicine in 1998. She was appointed to the Board of Directors of the American College for the Advancement of Medicine, where she currently serves as advisor to the board of directors. Through ACAM, she developed an integrative medicine boot camp for practitioners and their first webinar-based chelation therapy workshop. In addition, she is on the Scientific Advisory Board of the Organic and Natural Health Association and of Cure Hydration.

In 2018 Cohen co-authored *Quench* with Gina Bria, which garnered rave reviews and has a cult following. Cohen also performed in the off-Broadway show *The Thinnest Woman with the Fewest Wrinkles Wins*, a meditation on body image, weight issues, and plastic surgery. She spends weekends in the Hudson Valley with her husband, Henry, and their dog, Frida. On weekdays, Frida can often be found in the office greeting patients.

FuelUp

Colin Sapire is the founder and CEO of Beast Health®, and a titan in the world of blending. Driven by a passion for nutrition, Sapire revolutionized the blender industry as the co-founder and former CEO of Nutribullet®, LLC.* He kickstarted the personal blending category with the introduction of the NutriBullet®, and turned it into a kitchen staple in millions of homes. In 2021, Sapire launched Beast Health as an all-encompassing wellness brand on a mission to elevate the blending experience and encourage people to increase their consumption of nature's foods. Beast's flagship product, the viral, award-winning Beast Blender, is a premium personal blender that looks beautiful on your countertop and performs unlike any other blender on the market.

As a lifelong marathon runner, Colin's passion for blending began as a solution to his own nutrition struggles. He'd always been a steak and fries kind of guy, but needed a way to increase his intake of whole foods and nutrients in order to optimize his health and meet the mental and physical demands of his career and athletic pursuits. So, he began blending and drinking a green smoothie composed entirely of vegetables every morning. In doing this, he realized that for many people like himself, blending could be an exceptional, life-changing health unlock. With no time to cook, and a disdain for the taste of salads and "healthy" foods, Colin was able to transform his nutrition, and improve his energy levels, health, and overall well-being by starting each day with a nutrient-packed green blend. The only headache was the large, clunky, old-school blender he was using to blend each morning. And thus, the personal blender was born!

As the personal blending revolution took hold, Sapire began spearheading wellness initiatives within the brand, including a public school nutrition program and a marathon training and running team. After selling Nutribullet in 2018, Sapire embarked on his next mission: elevate personal blending and create tools to inspire a new generation of more mindful, quality-focused consumers to live a healthier lifestyle. With cutting-edge design and patented safety features, the Beast Blender became a favorite among celebrities like Oprah and Halle Berry, and publications like *Forbes, Financial Times,* and *Consumer Reports,* and has won several global design awards and is now beloved in homes around the world.

*Nutribullet® is the registered trademark of Capbran Holdings, LLC.

Born in South Africa, Colin currently resides in Los Angeles, California, where he maintains an extensive garden of fruit trees, vegetables, herbs, and edible flowers that he adds to his blends daily. He continues to make a "green slime" blend every morning, but now he does so in style.

Resources and Recommendations

Find and Follow Us!

For more information about our work, go to:
Beast Health: TheBeast.com
Instagram: @BeastHealth
Facebook: @BeastHealth
YouTube: @BeastHealth
Dr. Dana Cohen: DrDanaCohen.com
Instagram: @DrDanaCohen
Facebook: @DanaCohenMD
YouTube: @DrDanaCohen

Blending Tips and Tricks

Blenders create heat, but I want my blend cold!

Blenders create friction as they break down food, which can create a little heat. Most of us like our smoothies and other blends cold, so an easy way to keep them nice and chilly is to add ice or use frozen ingredients.

How to achieve the perfect texture.

Adding ice to your smoothies will not only make them cold; it will also make them thick and slushy. Alternatively (or in addition), you can use frozen ingredients. Most smoothie ingredients freeze quite nicely, including bananas, berries, greens, and protein options like peas and edamame. And you will always be smoothie ready when you have frozen ingredients on hand.

Don't put hot stuff in your blender.

Hot ingredients can expand while blending, creating an environment that can damage your blender or worse, cause injury. Always let ingredients get to room temperature before blending. For recipes like soups, sauces, and stews, use cold or room-temperature ingredients in the blender, then heat in a pot on the stove.

Sometimes things don't go perfectly when we blend.

Some ingredients are tougher than others or don't blend exactly as planned, leaving behind unblended chunks. If that happens, or your blender gets caught up, take the vessel off the base and give the ingredients a shake to move things around. If that doesn't help, add some liquid and give it another good shake, or stir with a spoon, before blending again.

Don't overfill your blender.

Pay attention to the max line on your blender; it's there for a reason! Your blender needs room for the ingredients to move around and the blades to spin, creating turbulence. When you overfill it, your blender will struggle to provide you with the perfect texture. If you find you have too much in your blender, stop blending, remove some of the contents, and start again.

Pay special attention to nuts, seeds, and powders.

It's best to have small ingredients like chia seeds, nuts, and protein powder next to the blade so they get broken down and don't create clumps. Every smoothie recipe in this book was created using the Beast blender. For best results when using this kind of personal blender, load your blender by following the order of the ingredients in the recipe. Always start with your liquid and then add the remaining ingredients in the order they appear. For other types of blenders, consult the manual for the optimal loading order.

Cleaning tips

Blenders are really easy to clean if you rinse them out right away, before the ingredients dry! Even if you don't have time to fully wash your vessel, give it a rinse so you don't have to deal with dried, stuck-on ingredients later on. (For more cleaning tips, see page 28.)

The Best of the Beast®

Like we said early on in this book, healthy habits are more sustainable if they are easy and enjoyable. That's why we are including a shameless plug for the Beast blender. In our humble opinion, it makes *Fueling Up* that much better for a variety of reasons.

First, the Beast blender is unlike any other personal blender. With aesthetic beauty, superior craftsmanship, and premium materials, the Beast offers best-in-class engineering and performance so you get a silky-smooth, mouthwatering blend every time.

The Beast is:

- So attractive you leave it on your countertop, reminding you to use it.

- So quick and easy, it fits into your busy day.

- So powerful it blends tough ingredients like ginger and celery until they are silky smooth and delicious.

Power and Precision

The Beast's motors are tuned for maximum performance and can be controlled by a single, highly responsive button to pulse and blend with precision.

Secure Connection

The Beast's industry-leading electronic interlock system confirms that the vessel, blade assembly, and blender base are all securely connected before it begins blending.

Silky-Smooth Blends

The innovative 12-rib vessel design of the Beast creates increased turbulence and blending efficiency . . . and the smoothest blends.

Temperature Sensor

The Beast's patented thermal safety sensor will automatically shut off if the ingredients get too hot.

Protein Powders

We prefer to use whole foods from nature in our blends, but protein powder can be a convenient alternative to help ensure you are getting the protein you need. However, all brands are not created equal. Some are filled with the same kinds of sweeteners, fillers, and artificial ingredients that are often in UPFs, so make sure to check labels before you buy.

There are many types of protein powders available. Here is a breakdown to help you find one that is right for you.

Pea Protein

If you are looking for a plant-based protein, pea protein is made from dried, ground-up peas. Unlike other plant proteins, pea contains all nine of the essential amino acids our bodies need.

Whey Protein

Often used by athletes and bodybuilders, whey protein is animal based and extracted from milk. The process separates the protein from casein and fat but includes all nine essential amino acids.

Rice Protein

A plant-based option that is a rich source of protein but doesn't contain all nine essential amino acids, this is okay if you are getting other sources of protein throughout the day.

Hydrolyzed Beef Protein

A popular choice for Paleo eaters, this beef-based protein is created by boiling beef down to a liquid and skimming the protein away from the carbohydrates and fat. It's a rich source of protein and contains all nine essential amino acids, but it has been shown to be less bioavailable than whey protein.

You are welcome to choose your favorite protein powder brand, of course, but if you are looking for a trusted source, Dr. Dana recommends the following options, which you can find on her website, DrDanaCohen.com:

InflammaQuench: A protein powder blend with 19 grams of protein per serving, which also includes nutrients to address immune challenges, maintain normal inflammatory balance, and strengthen gastrointestinal barrier function. Offered in vanilla chai or strawberry flavors.

CarbQuench: A protein powder blend with 10 grams of protein per serving, which also includes nutrients to support blood sugar balance. Offered in chocolate or vanilla flavors.

NutraQuench: A strawberry-flavored protein blend with 15 grams of protein per serving, which also includes nutrients to help recharge cellular energy production, increase antioxidant protection, support detoxification capacity, and support immune function. Better than a multivitamin!

Other supplemental powders from Dr. Dana include:

GreenQuench: A greens powder combining concentrated, organic fruits and berries with a vegetable antioxidant blend for those who have trouble meeting their daily requirements through food.

BiomeQuench: A probiotic powder with a carefully assembled cast of probiotic organisms to support microflora balance and maintain a healthy environment.

CollagenQuench: A collagen powder that can be mixed into water or other liquids to provide concentrated bioactive collagen peptides taken to support cartilage, tendons, ligaments, fascia, bone, and skin.

MagQuench: A strawberry-lemonade–flavored reacted magnesium powder mix delivering 300 milligrams of magnesium bisglycinate chelate for the many Americans who fail to meet their daily requirement through food.

Shopping Guide

A great way to eat more as-nature-intended foods, and particularly more plants, is to shop your local farmer's markets or get farm-fresh food delivered through a community-supported agriculture (CSA) program. Use the following links to find ones near you:

Farmer's Market Places: Find one near you at farmersmarkeplaces.com.

LocalHarvest: Find CSAs, farms, and farmer's markets near you at localharvest.org.

Following are some more of our favorite shopping resources for groceries and growing kits so you can grow a few healthy options at home. Many of them are available via mail order throughout the country:

AeroGarden, aerogarden.com

Indoor hydroponic garden systems complete with LED grow lights and seed kits for herbs, salad greens, and even veggies like tomatoes and peppers.

Butcher Box, butcherbox.com

Online resource for quality meat and wild-caught seafood.

Costco, costco.com

A reasonably priced resource for all sorts of healthy foods—and some not-so-healthy foods too, so read those labels!

Hamama, hamama.com
Seed quilts and supplies to grow your own microgreens at home.
Northwest Wild Foods, nwwildfoods.com
A good source for aronia berries, frozen or dried, as well as other wild berries, nuts, mushrooms, and more.
Thrive, thrivemarket.com
A mail-order resource for groceries, including a variety of meat, fish, frozen foods, and nonperishables.
White Oak Pastures, whiteoakpastures.com
A family farm in Georgia focused on humane animal husbandry and zero-waste production that offers a wide variety of meats for home delivery.
Wild Alaskan Company, wildalaskancompany.com
A delivery resource for wild-caught, sustainable seafood.

Elimination Diet Information

When one of her patients suspects they have a food intolerance, Dr. Dana often recommends a simple elimination diet to test their reactions to the five most likely culprits. In her experience, the following foods account for more than 75 percent of all food intolerances:

- Dairy
- Gluten
- Eggs
- Corn
- Soy

To begin, eliminate all five foods from your diet for 21 days. After that time, methodically reintroduce one food at a time by eating it every day for 3 days.

If after 3 days, you have not experienced any symptoms, then move on to the next food. The one exception is dairy: Dr. Dana suggests reintroducing sheep's milk, goat's milk, and cow's milk products separately. In her experience, people who have problems with one kind of dairy can sometimes tolerate others.

For further information and suggestions, go to health.clevelan-clinic.org/elimination-diet. It's also a good idea to consult a dietitian or doctor before starting an elimination diet, especially if you experience pronounced symptoms or if this simple diet doesn't pinpoint the cause.

Sources for Finding a Holistic Practitioner

American College for Advancement in Medicine: www.acam.org
The Institute for Functional Medicine: www.ifm.org
Functional Medicine Coaching Academy:
www.directory.functionalmedicinecoaching.org

30 Plant Challenge: Surprising Foods That Count

When people think about adding plants to their diet, they often think about the obvious fruits and vegetables. Those are great options, of course, but there are a lot more options than that, some of which you may be overlooking. As you fill in the 30 Plant Challenge worksheet that follows, remember that everything on this list also counts!

Alliums like onions, garlic, leeks, shallots, scallions, and chives

Fermented plants like kimchi, sauerkraut, and natto

Herbs, dried or fresh, like mint, oregano, basil, lemongrass, dill, and rosemary

Spices like cinnamon, chili powder, mustard seeds or powder, paprika, and cumin

Black pepper

Nuts
Nut butters
Seeds like poppy, sesame, sunflower, flax, or hemp
Seed butters or pastes like tahini

Beans, dried or canned
Chickpeas: Whole ones count, of course, but also when blended to make hummus
Lentils
Split peas

Whole grains like oats, buckwheat, barley, farro, quinoa, and rice

Coffee

Chocolate

Mushrooms: While technically a fungus, they are rich in nutrients like plants are, so we think they should count.

Teas: Tea blends may even count as more than one plant. A typical chai-spice mix, for example, may contain black tea leaves, cinnamon, ginger, cardamom, cloves, and coriander. That's six plants!

Worksheets

30 Plant Challenge Worksheet + Hydration Status Tracker

Keep this chart in your kitchen so you can record all the different plants you eat as you eat them. Then tally them up at the end of the week!

You can use the final column to track your hydration status like we discussed in Chapter 4. Mark it down every time you urinate and then add up the marks at the end of each day. Remember that you want to be urinating every 2 to 3 hours while you're awake.

FuelUp

	Fruit Ex: berries, melons, apple	Vegetables Ex: leafy greens, root veggies	Herbs & Spices Ex: dried or fresh thyme, cinnamon	Nuts & Seeds Ex: walnuts, sesame seeds
Monday				
Tuesday				
Wednesday				
Thursday				
Friday				
Saturday				
Sunday				
Totals (Tally items in each column)	Total Weekly Fruits:	Total Weekly Veggies:	Total Weekly Herbs & Spices:	Total Weekly Nuts & Seeds:

Add together the numbers in the
bottom row to arrive at your Weekly Total: _____

Beans & Legumes Ex: lentils, peas, chickpeas	Whole Grains Ex: oats, farro, buckwheat, rice	Others Ex: teas, coffee, mushrooms	Urination Tracker
Total Weekly Beans & Legumes:	Total Weekly Grains:	Total Weekly Others:	

*Congratulations on consuming
such a wide variety of plants!*

7-Day Beast Blending Lifestyle Plan Meal Chart

Fill in the chart using our recipes or by making your own dishes using our Fuel Up Meal formula in Chapter 6.

	Breakfast Blends	Fuel Up Lunch	Fuel Up Dinner	Snack & Dessert Options (if desired)
Monday				
Tuesday				
Wednesday				
Thursday				
Friday				
Saturday				
Sunday				

Notes

Introduction: Healthy Eating Shouldn't Be So Hard

1. Lee et al., "Adults Meeting Fruit and Vegetable Intake Recommendations—United States, 2019," *Morbidity and Mortality Weekly Report* 71, no. 1 (January 7, 2022): 1–9, https://doi.org/10.15585/mmwr.mm7101a1.

2. Lee et al., "Adults Meeting Fruit and Vegetable Intake Recommendations."

3. Diane Quagliani and Patricia Felt-Gunderson, "Closing America's Fiber Intake Gap: Communication Strategies from a Food and Fiber Summit," *American Journal of Lifestyle Medicine* 11, no. 1 (2017): 80–5, https://doi.org/10.1177/1559827615588079.

4. Pickering et al., "Magnesium Status and Stress: The Vicious Circle Concept Revisited," *Nutrients* 12, no. 12 (2020): 3672, https://doi.org/10.3390/nu12123672.

5. Carlo Selmi and Koichi Tsuneyama, "Nutrition, Geoepidemiology, and Autoimmunity," *Autoimmunity Reviews* 9, no. 5 (March 2010): A267–70, https://doi.org/10.1016/j.autrev.2009.12.001.

6. Wallace et al., "Fruits, Vegetables, and Health: A Comprehensive Narrative, Umbrella Review of the Science and Recommendations for Enhanced Public Policy to Improve Intake," *Critical Reviews in Food Science and Nutrition* 60, no. 13 (2020): 2174–211, https://doi.org/10.1080/10408398.2019.1632258.

7. Downer et al., "Food Is Medicine: Actions to Integrate Food and Nutrition into Healthcare," *BMJ* 369 (2020): m2482, https://doi.org/10.1136/bmj.m2482.

8. Ferrer-Cascales et al., "Higher Adherence to the Mediterranean Diet Is Related to More Subjective Happiness in Adolescents: The Role of Health-Related Quality of Life," *Nutrients* 11, no. 3 (2019): 698, https://doi.org/10.3390/nu11030698.

9. Andrew Steptoe, "Happiness and Health," *Annual Review of Public Health* 40, no. 1 (2019): 339–59, https://doi.org/10.1146/annurev-publhealth-040218-044150.

10. Karl Peltzer and Supa Pengpid, "Dietary Consumption and Happiness and Depression among University Students: A Cross-National Survey," *Journal*

of Psychology in Africa 27, no. 4 (2017): 372–77, https://doi.org/10.108
0/14330237.2017.1347761.

11. "Consumers Plan to Eat Healthier in 2022," www.QSRweb.com, June
     20, 2023, accessed January 28, 2024, https://www.qsrweb.com/news/
     consumers-plan-to-eat-healthier-in-2022/.

12. Lee et al., "Adults Meeting Fruit and Vegetable Intake Recommendations."

13. "Fiber: The Carb That Helps You Manage Diabetes," Centers for Disease Control
     and Prevention, June 20, 2022, accessed January 21, 2023, https://www.cdc.gov/
     diabetes/library/features/role-of-fiber.html.

14. McDonald et al., "American Gut: An Open Platform for Citizen Science
     Microbiome Research," *MSystems* 3, no. 3 (2018), https://doi.org/10.1128/
     msystems.00031-18.

15. L. Fernando Reyes, J. Emilio Villarreal, and Luis Cisneros-Zevallos, "The Increase in
     Antioxidant Capacity after Wounding Depends on the Type of Fruit or Vegetable
     Tissue," *Food Chemistry* 101, no. 3 (2007): 1254–62, https://doi.org/10.1016/j
     .foodchem.2006.03.032.

16. Hu et al., "Biosynthesis of Phenolic Compounds and Antioxidant Activity in Fresh-
     Cut Fruits and Vegetables," *Frontiers in Microbiology* 13 (May 2022): 906069, https://
     doi.org/10.3389/fmicb.2022.906069.

17. Andrew Tatarsky, "Harm Reduction Psychotherapy: Extending the Reach of
     Traditional Substance Use Treatment," *Journal of Substance Abuse Treatment* 25, no.
     4 (December 2003): 249–56, https://doi.org/10.1016/s0740-5472(03)00085-0.

18. G. Alan Marlatt, ed., *Harm Reduction: Pragmatic Strategies for Managing High-Risk
     Behaviors* (New York: Guilford Press, 1998), P277.

19. San Diego State University, "Professors Examine What Influences Healthy,
     Sustainable Food Choices," ScienceDaily, September 11, 2019, accessed January 28,
     2024, https://www.sciencedaily.com/releases/2019/09/190911142725.htm.

Chapter 1: Make Blending a Habit

1. Mark 8:22–26 (NIV).

2. Luke 9:10–17 (NIV).

3. Katherine Wright, "The Origins and Development of Ground Stone Assemblages
    in Late Pleistocene Southwest Asia," *Paléorient* 17, no. 1 (1991): 19–45, https://doi.
    org/10.3406/paleo.1991.4537.

4. K. Aleisha Fetters, "Can You Really Learn to like Healthy Foods?," U.S. News &
    World Report, March 18, 2016, accessed January 31, 2024, https://health.usnews.
    com/wellness/articles/2016-03-18/can-you-really-learn-to-like-healthy-foods.

5. Philippa Heath, Carmel Houston-Price, and Orla B. Kennedy, "Increasing Food Familiarity without the Tears. A Role for Visual Exposure?," *Appetite* 57, no. 3 (December 2011): 832–38, https://doi.org/10.1016/j.appet.2011.05.315.

6. University of Pennsylvania, "Evolution of Bitter Taste Sensitivity," ScienceDaily, November 13, 2013, accessed January 31, 2024, https://www.sciencedaily.com/releases/2013/11/131111185522.htm.

7. Rezaie et al., "Effects of Bitter Substances on GI Function, Energy Intake and Glycaemia—Do Preclinical Findings Translate to Outcomes in Humans?," *Nutrients* 13, no. 4 (2021): 1317, https://doi.org/10.3390/nu13041317.

8. Elizabeth D. Capaldi-Phillips and Devina Wadhera, "Associative Conditioning Can Increase Liking for and Consumption of Brussels Sprouts in Children Aged 3 to 5 Years," *Journal of the Academy of Nutrition and Dietetics* 114, no. 8 (August 2014): 1236–41, https://doi.org/10.1016/j.jand.2013.11.014.

9. Tara Parker-Pope, "To Start a New Habit, Make It Easy," *New York Times*, January 9, 2021, Well|Mind section, accessed January 31, 2024, https://www.nytimes.com/2021/01/09/well/mind/healthy-habits.html.

10. Yang et al., "Effectiveness of Commercial and Homemade Washing Agents in Removing Pesticide Residues on and in Apples," Journal of Agricultural and Food Chemistry 65, no. 44 (October 2017): 9744–52, https://doi.org/10.1021/acs.jafc.7b03118.

11. Thich Nhat Hanh, *How to Eat* (TK City: National Geographic Books, 2014).

12. "Loneliness and Social Isolation Linked to Serious Health Conditions," Centers for Disease Control and Prevention, n.d., accessed November 6, 2023, https://www.cdc.gov/aging/publications/features/lonely-older-adults.html.

13. Bédard et al., "Can Eating Pleasure Be a Lever for Healthy Eating? A Systematic Scoping Review of Eating Pleasure and Its Links with Dietary Behaviors and Health," *PLoS ONE* 15, no. 12 (December 21, 2020): e0244292, https://doi.org/10.1371/journal.pone.0244292.

14. Simone Pettigrew, "Pleasure: An Under-Utilised 'P' in Social Marketing for Healthy Eating," *Appetite* 104 (September 1, 2016): 60–9, https://doi.org/10.1016/j.appet.2015.10.004.

Chapter 2: Consume More Foods as Nature Intended

1. Juul et al., "Ultra-Processed Food Consumption and Excess Weight among US Adults," *British Journal of Nutrition* 120, no. 1 (May 6, 2018): 90–100, https://doi.org/10.1017/s0007114518001046.

2. Ares et al., "Consumers' Conceptualization of Ultra-Processed Foods," *Appetite* 105 (October 1, 2016): 611–17, https://doi.org/10.1016/j.appet.2016.06.028.

3. Anahad O'Connor and Aaron Steckelberg, "Melted, Pounded, Extruded: Why Many Ultra-Processed Foods Are Unhealthy," *Washington Post,* June 28, 2023, Well+Being section, accessed November 26, 2023, https://www.washingtonpost.com/wellness/2023/06/27/ultra-processed-foods-predigested-health-risks/.

4. Chen et al., "Consumption of Ultra-Processed Foods and Health Outcomes: A Systematic Review of Epidemiological Studies," *Nutrition Journal* 19 (2020): no. 86, https://doi.org/10.1186/s12937-020-00604-1.

5. "Jerry Seinfeld Interview: How to Write a Joke," *New York Times,* December 20, 2012, YouTube video, https://www.youtube.com/watch?v=itWxXyCfW5s.

6. Pagliai et al., "Consumption of Ultra-Processed Foods and Health Status: A Systematic Review and Meta-Analysis," *British Journal of Nutrition* 125, no. 3 (August 14, 2020): 308–18, https://doi.org/10.1017/s0007114520002688.

7. Elizabeth et al., "Ultra-Processed Foods and Health Outcomes: A Narrative Review," *Nutrients* 12, no. 7 (2020): 1955, https://doi.org/10.3390/nu12071955.

8. David Basic and Christopher Shanley, "Frailty in an Older Inpatient Population: Using the Clinical Frailty Scale to Predict Patient Outcomes," *Journal of Aging and Health* 27, no. 4 (2015): 670–85, https://doi.org/10.1177/0898264314558202.

9. Gonçalves et al., "Association between Consumption of Ultraprocessed Foods and Cognitive Decline," *JAMA Neurology* 80, no. 2 (2023): 142–50, https://doi.org/10.1001/jamaneurol.2022.4397.

10. Pagliai et al., "Consumption of Ultra-Processed Foods and Health Status."

11. Schiestl et al., "A Narrative Review of Highly Processed Food Addiction across the Lifespan," *Progress in Neuro-Psychopharmacology and Biological Psychiatry* 106 (March 2021): 110152, https://doi.org/10.1016/j.pnpbp.2020.110152.

12. Ashley N. Gearhardt and Johannes Hebebrand, "The Concept of 'Food Addiction' Helps Inform the Understanding of Overeating and Obesity: Debate Consensus," *The American Journal of Clinical Nutrition* 113, no. 2 (February 2021): 274–76, https://doi.org/10.1093/ajcn/nqaa345.

13. Chassaing et al., "Dietary Emulsifiers Directly Alter Human Microbiota Composition and Gene Expression Ex Vivo Potentiating Intestinal Inflammation," *Gut* 66, no. 8 (2017): 1414–27, https://doi.org/10.1136/gutjnl-2016-313099.

14. Bénard et al., "Degraded Carrageenan Causing Colitis in Rats Induces TNF Secretion and ICAM-1 Upregulation in Monocytes through NF-κB Activation," *PLoS ONE* 5, no. 1 (January 2010): e8666, https://doi.org/10.1371/journal.pone.0008666.

15. Juul et al., "Ultra-Processed Food Consumption among US Adults from 2001 to 2018," *The American Journal of Clinical Nutrition* 115, no. 1 (January 2022): 211–21, https://doi.org/10.1093/ajcn/nqab305.

16. Baraldi et al., "Consumption of Ultra-Processed Foods and Associated Sociodemographic Factors in the USA between 2007 and 2012: Evidence from a

Nationally Representative Cross-Sectional Study," *BMJ Open* 8 (2018): e020574, https://doi.org/10.1136/bmjopen-2017-020574.

17. Gupta et al., "Characterizing Ultra-Processed Foods by Energy Density, Nutrient Density, and Cost," *Frontiers in Nutrition* 6 (May 2019), https://doi.org/10.3389/fnut.2019.00070.

18. Juul et al., "Ultra-Processed Food Consumption among US Adults."

19. Monteiro et al., "The UN Decade of Nutrition, the NOVA Food Classification and the Trouble with Ultra-Processing," *Public Health Nutrition* 21, no. 1 (March 2017): 5–17, https://doi.org/10.1017/s1368980017000234.

20. "Trans Fats," www.heart.org, March 23, 2017, accessed January 25, 2024, https://www.heart.org/en/healthy-living/healthy-eating/eat-smart/fats/trans-fat.

21. Remig et al., "*Trans* Fats in America: A Review of Their Use, Consumption, Health Implications, and Regulation," *Journal of the Academy of Nutrition and Dietetics* 110, no. 4 (April 2010): 585–92, https://doi.org/10.1016/j.jada.2009.12.024.

22. Center for Food Safety and Applied Nutrition, "Food Labeling & Nutrition," U.S. Food and Drug Administration, December 13, 2023, accessed January 25, 2024, https://www.fda.gov/food/food-labeling-nutrition.

23. John Kell, "What Campbell Learned from a 101-Year-Old Tomato Soup Recipe," *Fortune*, December 19, 2016, accessed December 15, 2023, https://fortune.com/2016/12/19/campbell-soup-old-soup-recipe/.

24. Peter Williams, "Consumer Understanding and Use of Health Claims for Foods," *Nutrition Reviews* 63, no. 7 (July 2005): 256–64, https://doi.org/10.1111/j.1753-4887.2005.tb00382.x.

25. Colby et al., "Nutrition Marketing on Food Labels," *Journal of Nutrition Education and Behavior* 42, no. 2 (March 2010): 92–8, https://doi.org/10.1016/j.jneb.2008.11.002.

26. Center for Food Safety and Applied Nutrition, "Use of the Term Natural on Food Labeling," U.S. Food and Drug Administration, October 22, 2018, accessed February 6, 2024, https://www.fda.gov/food/food-labeling-nutrition/use-term-natural-food-labeling.

27. USDA Agricultural Marketing Service, "What Is Organic?," U.S. Department of Agriculture, n.d., September 1, 2011, accessed February 6, 2024, https://www.ams.usda.gov/publications/content/what-organic.

28. Vigar et al., "A Systematic Review of Organic versus Conventional Food Consumption: Is There a Measurable Benefit on Human Health?" *Nutrients* 12, no. 1 (2020): 7, https://doi.org/10.3390/nu12010007.

29. Jennifer Leake, "Ultra-Processed Foods: Why Did We Create Them and Why Can't We Stop Eating Them?," ABC Listen, November 11, 2023, accessed January 28, 2024, https://www.abc.net.au/listen/programs/rearvision/what-makes-food-ultra-processed-and-why-they-make-us-eat-more/102961240.

30. Stephanie Eckelkamp, "You're Tossing One of the Healthiest Parts of Your Watermelon—Stop!" *Prevention*, July 12, 2016, accessed February 6, 2024, https://www.prevention.com/food-nutrition/healthy-eating/a20437529/watermelon-rind-nutrition/.

Chapter 3: Variety Variety Variety

1. Center for Food Safety and Applied Nutrition, "Daily Value on the Nutrition and Supplement Facts Labels," U.S. Food and Drug Administration, September 27, 2023, accessed June 29, 2023, https://www.fda.gov/food/new-nutrition-facts-label/daily-value-new-nutrition-and-supplement-facts-labels.

2. Thompson et al., "Association of Healthful Plant-Based Diet Adherence with Risk of Mortality and Major Chronic Diseases among Adults in the UK." *JAMA Network Open* 6, no. 3 (March 2023): e234714, https://doi.org/10.1001/jamanetworkopen.2023.4714.

3. National Institutes of Health Office of Dietary Supplements, "Potassium: Fact Sheet for Health Professionals," National Institutes of Health, n.d., accessed December 23, 2023, https://ods.od.nih.gov/factsheets/Potassium-HealthProfessional/.

4. National Institutes of Health Office of Dietary Supplements, "Vitamin E: Fact Sheet for Health Professionals," National Institutes of Health, n.d., accessed January 27, 2024, https://ods.od.nih.gov/factsheets/VitaminE-HealthProfessional/.

5. Tyler R. Kemnic, "Vitamin E Deficiency." In book: *StatPearls* [Internet] (Treasure Island, FL: StatPearls Publishing, 2023), https://www.ncbi.nlm.nih.gov/books/NBK519051/.

6. Reider et al., "Inadequacy of Immune Health Nutrients: Intakes in US Adults, the 2005–2016 NHANES." *Nutrients* 12, no. 6 (2020): 1735, https://doi.org/10.3390/nu12061735.

7. U.S. Department of Agriculture and U.S. Department of Health and Human Services, *Dietary Guidelines for Americans: 2020–2025*, 9th ed., https://www.dietaryguidelines.gov/sites/default/files/2021-03/Dietary_Guidelines_for_Americans-2020-2025.pdf.

8. Jennifer Di Noia, "Defining Powerhouse Fruits and Vegetables: A Nutrient Density Approach," *Preventing Chronic Disease* 11 (June 5, 2014): 130290, https://doi.org/10.5888/pcd11.130390.

9. Morris et al., "Nutrients and Bioactives in Green Leafy Vegetables and Cognitive Decline," *Neurology* 90, no. 3 (January 16, 2018), https://doi.org/10.1212/wnl.0000000000004815.https://www.cdc.gov/diabetes/php/data-research/?CDC_AAref_Val=https://www.cdc.gov/diabetes/data/statistics-report/index.htmld Order Has a Significant Impact on Postprandial Glucose and Insulin Levels," *Diabetes Care* 38, no. 7 (June 1, 2015): e98–9, https://doi.org/10.2337/dc15-0429.

10. "National Diabetes Statistics Report," Centers for Disease Control and Prevention, n.d., accessed December 14, 2023, https://www.cdc.gov/diabetes/data/statistics-report/index.html.

NOTES

11. Noad et al., "Beneficial Effect of a Polyphenol-Rich Diet on Cardiovascular Risk: A Randomised Control Trial," *Heart* 102, no. 17 (2016): 1371–9, https://doi.org/10.1136/heartjnl-2015-309218.

12. Del Bo' et al., "Systematic Review on Polyphenol Intake and Health Outcomes: Is There Sufficient Evidence to Define a Health-Promoting Polyphenol-Rich Dietary Pattern?" *Nutrients* 11, no. 6 (2019): 1355, https://doi.org/10.3390/nu11061355.

13. Liu et al., "Relationship between Dietary Polyphenols and Gut Microbiota: New Clues to Improve Cognitive Disorders, Mood Disorders and Circadian Rhythms," *Foods* 12, no. 6 (2023): 1309, https://doi.org/10.3390/foods12061309.

14. Noad et al., "Beneficial Effect of a Polyphenol-Rich Diet." Giuseppe Grosso, "Effects of Polyphenol-Rich Foods on Human Health," *Nutrients* 10, no. 8 (2018): 1089, https://doi.org/10.3390/nu10081089.

15. Del Bo' et al., "Systematic Review on Polyphenol Intake." USDA Economic Research Service, "Food Availability and Consumption," U.S. Department of Agriculture, n.d., accessed July 2, 2023, https://www.ers.usda.gov/data-products/ag-and-food-statistics-charting-the-essentials/food-availability-and-consumption/.

16. Harold McGee, *On Food and Cooking: The Science and Lore of the Kitchen* (New York: Scribner, 2004).

17. Cheng et al., "Lycopene and Tomato and Risk of Cardiovascular Diseases: A Systematic Review and Meta-Analysis of Epidemiological Evidence," *Critical Reviews in Food Science and Nutrition* 59, no. 1 (2019): 141–58, https://doi.org/10.1080/10408398.2017.1362630.

18. Li et al., "Tomato and Lycopene and Multiple Health Outcomes: Umbrella Review," *Food Chemistry* 343 (May 2021): 128396, https://doi.org/10.1016/j.foodchem.2020.128396.

19. P. W. Simon, "Carrot Facts," U.S. Department of Agriculture, n.d., accessed June 30, 2023, https://www.ars.usda.gov/midwest-area/madison-wi/vegetable-crops-research/docs/simon-carrot-facts/.

20. P. W. Simon, "Pigment Power in Carrot Colors: How Pigments Promote Good Health," U.S. Department of Agriculture, n.d., accessed June 30, 2023, https://www.ars.usda.gov/midwest-area/madison-wi/vegetable-crops-research/docs/simon-pigment-power/.

21. U.S. Department of Agriculture and U.S. Department of Health and Human Services, *Dietary Guidelines for Americans, 2020–2025.*

22. Diane Quagliani and Patricia Felt-Gunderson, "Closing America's Fiber Intake Gap: Communication Strategies from a Food and Fiber Summit," *American Journal of Lifestyle Medicine* 11, no. 1 (2017): 80–5. Accessed June 30, 2023. https://doi.org/10.1177/1559827615588079.

23. Kevin B. Miller, "Review of Whole Grain and Dietary Fiber Recommendations and Intake Levels in Different Countries," *Nutrition Reviews* 78, Supplement 1 (July 30, 2020): 29–36, https://doi.org/10.1093/nutrit/nuz052.

24. Harvard Health Publishing, "The Good Side of Bacteria," Harvard Medical School, April 7, 2023, accessed June 23, 2023, https://www.health.harvard.edu/staying-healthy/the-good-side-of-bacteria.

25. Makki et al., "The Impact of Dietary Fiber on Gut Microbiota in Host Health and Disease," *Cell Host & Microbe* 23, no. 6 (June 13, 2018): 705–15, https://doi.org/10.1016/j.chom.2018.05.012.

26. Oh et al., "A Universal Gut-Microbiome-Derived Signature Predicts Cirrhosis," *Cell Metabolism* 32, no. 5 (November 3, 2020): 878—88.E6, https://doi.org/10.1016/j.cmet.2020.06.005.

27. Blanco-Pérez et al., "The Dietary Fiber Pectin: Health Benefits and Potential for the Treatment of Allergies by Modulation of Gut Microbiota," *Current Allergy and Asthma Reports* 21, no. 43 (2021), https://doi.org/10.1007/s11882-021-01020-z.

28. Katerina V. A. Johnson, "Gut Microbiome Composition and Diversity Are Related to Human Personality Traits," *Human Microbiome Journal* 15 (March 2020): 100069, https://doi.org/10.1016/j.humic.2019.100069.

29. Sumich et al., "Gut Microbiome-Brain Axis and Inflammation in Temperament, Personality and Psychopathology," *Current Opinion in Behavioral Sciences* 44 (April 2022): 101101, https://doi.org/10.1016/j.cobeha.2022.101101.

30. Vernice et al., "The Gut Microbiome and Psycho-Cognitive Traits," In *Progress in Molecular Biology and Translational Science* 176 (2020): 123–40, https://doi.org/10.1016/bs.pmbts.2020.08.014.

31. Marco et al., "Health Benefits of Fermented Foods: Microbiota and Beyond," *Current Opinion in Biotechnology* 44 (April 2017): 94–102, https://doi.org/10.1016/j.copbio.2016.11.010.

32. Kojima et al., "Natto Intake Is Inversely Associated with Osteoporotic Fracture Risk in Postmenopausal Japanese Women," *The Journal of Nutrition* 150, no. 3 (March 2020): 599–605, https://doi.org/10.1093/jn/nxz292.

33. "What Is Resistant Starch?," The Johns Hopkins Patient Guide to Diabetes, n.d., accessed June 27, 2023, https://hopkinsdiabetesinfo.org/what-is-resistant-starch/.

34. McDonald et al., "American Gut: An Open Platform for Citizen Science Microbiome Research," *MSystems* 3, no. 3 (2018), https://doi.org/10.1128/msystems.00031-18.

35. Lee et al., "Adults Meeting Fruit and Vegetable Intake Recommendations—United States, 2019," *Morbidity and Mortality Weekly Report* 71, no. 1 (January 7, 2022): 1–9, https://doi.org/10.15585/mmwr.mm7101a1.

36. Mummah et al., "Effect of a Mobile App Intervention on Vegetable Consumption in Overweight Adults: A Randomized Controlled Trial," *International Journal of Behavioral Nutrition and Physical Activity* 14, no. 125 (2017), https://doi.org/10.1186/s12966-017-0563-2.

Chapter 4: Hydration as Fuel

1. Stookey et al., "Underhydration Is Associated with Obesity, Chronic Diseases, and Death Within 3 to 6 Years in the U.S. Population Aged 51–70 Years," *Nutrients* 12, no. 4 (2020): 905, https://doi.org/10.3390/nu12040905.

2. Dmitrieva et al., "Middle-Age High Normal Serum Sodium as a Risk Factor for Accelerated Biological Aging, Chronic Diseases, and Premature Mortality," *The Lancet* 87 (January 2023): 104404, https://doi.org/10.1016/j.ebiom.2022.104404.

3. "Link Between Hydration and Aging," National Institutes of Health, January 24, 2023, accessed November 27, 2023, https://www.nih.gov/news-events/nih-research-matters/link-between-hydration-aging.

4. Kostelnik et al., "The Validity of Urine Color as a Hydration Biomarker within the General Adult Population and Athletes: A Systematic Review," *Journal of the American College of Nutrition* 40, no. 2 (2021): 172–9, https://doi.org/10.1080/0731 5724.2020.1750073.

5. Andres-Hernando et al., "Vasopressin Mediates Fructose-Induced Metabolic Syndrome by Activating the V1b Receptor," *JCI Insight* 6, no. 1 (January 11, 2021): e140848, https://doi.org/10.1172/jci.insight.140848.

6. Rachel C. Vreeman and Aaron E. Carroll, "Medical Myths," *BMJ* 335 (2007): 1288, https://doi.org/10.1136/bmj.39420.420370.25.

7. Dana Benson, "Thirsty? You're Already Dehydrated," Baylor College of Medicine, August 9, 2021, accessed November 28, 2023, https://www.bcm.edu/news/thirsty-you-are-already-dehydrated.

8. Sagelv et al., "Device-Measured Physical Activity, Sedentary Time, and Risk of All-Cause Mortality: An Individual Participant Data Analysis of Four Prospective Cohort Studies," *British Journal of Sports Medicine* 57, no. 22 (2023): 1457–63, https://doi.org/10.1136/bjsports-2022-106568.

9. Ronald J. Maughan and James D. Griffin, "Caffeine Ingestion and Fluid Balance: A Review," *Journal of Human Nutrition and Dietetics* 16, no. 6 (2003): 411–20, https://pubmed.ncbi.nlm.nih.gov/19774754/#:~:text=Results%3A%20The%20available%20literature%20suggests,period%20of%20days%20or%20weeks.

10. Jessica Freeborn, "Low Salt Diet and Heart Failure: Surprising Findings on Life Quality, Hospitalization," Medical News Today, April 8, 2022, accessed November 27, 2023, https://www.medicalnewstoday.com/articles/low-salt-diet-and-heart-failure-surprising-findings-on-life-quality-hospitalization.

11. Li et al., "Salt Restriction and Risk of Adverse Outcomes in Heart Failure with Preserved Ejection Fraction," *Heart* 0 (July 18, 2022): 1–6, https://todayspractitioner.com/wp-content/uploads/2022/07/Salt-Restriction-and-Heart-Study.pdf.

Chapter 5: Play with Your Food

1. Adrian Furnham and K. V. Petrides, "Trait Emotional Intelligence and Happiness," *Social Behavior and Personality* 31, no. 8 (January 1, 2003): 815–23, https://doi.org/10.2224/sbp.2003.31.8.815.

2. "How Smell and Taste Change as You Age," National Institute on Aging, reviewed June 30, 2020, accessed September 20, 2023, https://www.nia.nih.gov/health/teeth-and-mouth/how-smell-and-taste-change-you-age#taste.

3. Yang et al., "Effect of Dietary Fiber on Constipation: A Meta Analysis," *World Journal of Gastroenterology* 18, no. 48 (2012): 7378–83, https://doi.org/10.3748/wjg.v18.i48.7378.

4. M. C. E. Lomer, "Review Article: The Aetiology, Diagnosis, Mechanisms and Clinical Evidence for Food Intolerance," *Alimentary Pharmacology & Therapeutics* 41, no. 3 (2015): 262–75, https://doi.org/10.1111/apt.13041.

5. Prashant Regmi and Leonie K. Heilbronn, "Time-Restricted Eating: Benefits, Mechanisms, and Challenges in Translation." *iScience* 23, no. 6 (June 26, 2020): 101161, https://doi.org/10.1016/j.isci.2020.101161.

6. Chaix et al., "Time-Restricted Eating to Prevent and Manage Chronic Metabolic Diseases," *Annual Review of Nutrition* 39 (2019): 291–315, https://doi.org/10.1146/annurev-nutr-082018-124320.

7. Armin Ezzati and Victoria M. Pak, "The Effects of Time-Restricted Eating on Sleep, Cognitive Decline, and Alzheimer's Disease," *Experimental Gerontology* 171 (January 2023): 112033, https://doi.org/10.1016/j.exger.2022.112033.

8. Chung et al., "Does the Proximity of Meals to Bedtime Influence the Sleep of Young Adults? A Cross-Sectional Survey of University Students," *International Journal of Environmental Research and Public Health* 17, no. 8 (2020): 2677, https://doi.org/10.3390/ijerph17082677.

9. Librairie Larousse, *Larousse Gastronomique: The World's Greatest Culinary Encyclopedia* (New York: Clarkson Potter Publishers, 2001).

10. Taheri et al., "Underutilized Chokeberry (*Aronia melanocarpa, Aronia arbutifolia, Aronia prunifolia*) Accessions Are Rich Sources of Anthocyanins, Flavonoids, Hydroxycinnamic Acids, and Proanthocyanidins." *Journal of Agricultural and Food Chemistry* 61, no. 36 (2013): 8581–88, https://doi.org/10.1021/jf402449q.

11. Jaramillo Flores et al., "Cocoa Flavanols: Natural Agents with Attenuating Effects on Metabolic Syndrome Risk Factors," *Nutrients* 11, no. 4 (2019): 751, https://doi.org/10.3390/nu11040751.

12. Miller et al., "Impact of Alkalization on the Antioxidant and Flavanol Content of Commercial Cocoa Powders," *Journal of Agricultural and Food Chemistry* 56, no. 18 (2008): 8527–33, https://doi.org/10.1021/jf801670p.

13. Frederic Rosengarten, *The Book of Spices* (New York: Pyramid Books, 1973).

14. Zare et al., "Efficacy of Cinnamon in Patients with Type II Diabetes Mellitus: A Randomized Controlled Clinical Trial," *Clinical Nutrition* 38, no. 2 (April 2019): 549–56, https://doi.org/10.1016/j.clnu.2018.03.003.

15. Souissi et al., "Antibacterial and Anti-Inflammatory Activities of Cardamom (*Elettaria cardamomum*) Extracts: Potential Therapeutic Benefits for Periodontal Infections," *Anaerobe* 61 (February 2020): 102089, https://doi.org/10.1016/j.anaerobe.2019.102089.

16. Betül Kocaadam and Nevin Şanlıer, "Curcumin, an Active Component of Turmeric (*Curcuma longa*), and Its Effects on Health," *Critical Reviews in Food Science and Nutrition* 57, no. 13 (2017): 2889–95, https://doi.org/10.1080/10408398.2015.1077195.

17. Haniadka et al., "A Review of the Gastroprotective Effects of Ginger (*Zingiber officinale Roscoe*)," *Food & Function* 4, no. 6 (2013): 845–55, https://doi.org/10.1039/c3fo30337c.

18. Coleman-Jensen et al., *Household Food Security in the United States in 2018*, U.S. Department of Agriculture Economic Research Service, September 2019, https://www.ers.usda.gov/webdocs/publications/94849/err-270.pdf?v=4680.8.

19. Serusha Govender, "These Countries Waste Enough Food to Feed the Planet," The Daily Meal, August 6, 2014, accessed September 27, 2023, https://www.thedailymeal.com/these-countries-waste-enough-food-feed-planet/.

20. Oliver Milman, "Americans Waste 150,000 Tons of Food Each Day—Equal to a Pound per Person," *Guardian*, April 18, 2018, Food section, accessed September 27, 2023, https://www.theguardian.com/environment/2018/apr/18/americans-waste-food-fruit-vegetables-study.

21. Emilio Ros, "Eat Nuts, Live Longer," *Journal of the American College of Cardiology* 70, no. 20 (November 2017): 2533–5, https://doi.org/10.1016/j.jacc.2017.09.1082.

22. Senizza et al., "Lignans and Gut Microbiota: An Interplay Revealing Potential Health Implications," *Molecules* 25, no. 23 (2020): 5709, https://doi.org/10.3390/molecules25235709.

23. J. M. Landete, "Plant and Mammalian Lignans: A Review of Source, Intake, Metabolism, Intestinal Bacteria and Health." *Food Research International* 46, no. 1 (April 2012): 410–24, https://doi.org/10.1016/j.foodres.2011.12.023.

Chapter 6: The 7-Day Beast Blending Lifestyle Plan

1. Mills et al., "Frequency of Eating Home Cooked Meals and Potential Benefits for Diet and Health: Cross-Sectional Analysis of a Population-Based Cohort Study," *International Journal of Behavioral Nutrition and Physical Activity* 14, no. 109 (2017), https://doi.org/10.1186/s12966-017-0567-y.

2. Qin et al., "Fried-Food Consumption and Risk of Cardiovascular Disease and All-Cause Mortality: A Meta-Analysis of Observational Studies," *Heart* 107, no. 19 (2021): 1567–75, https://doi.org/10.1136/heartjnl-2020-317883.

Hay House Titles of Related Interest

YOU CAN HEAL YOUR LIFE, the movie,
starring Louise Hay & Friends
(available as an online streaming video)
www.hayhouse.com/louise-movie

THE SHIFT, the movie,
starring Dr. Wayne W. Dyer
(available as an online streaming video)
www.hayhouse.com/the-shift-movie

***

BOUDNLESS KITCHEN: Biohack Your Body & Boost Your Brain with Healthy
Recipes You Actually Want to Eat, by Ben Greenfield

GROW A NEW BODY: How Spirit and Power Plant Nutrients
Can Transform Your Health, by Alberto Villoldo

HEALING ADAPTOGENS: The Definitive Guide to Using Super Herbs
and Mushrooms for Your Body's Restoration, Defense, and Performance,
by Tero Isokauppila and Danielle Ryan Broida

POSTDIABETIC: An Easy-to-Follow 9-Week Guide to Reversing Prediabetes
and Type 2 Diabetes, by Eric Edmeades and Ruben Ruiz, M.D.

REAL SUPERFOODS: Everyday Ingredients to Elevate Your Health,
by Ocean Robbins and Nichole Dandrea-Russert, MS, RDN

All of the above are available at your local bookstore or may be ordered by visiting:

Hay House USA: www.hayhouse.com
Hay House Australia: www.hayhouse.com.au
Hay House UK: www.hayhouse.co.uk
Hay House India: www.hayhouse.co.in

All of the above are available at your local bookstore,
or may be ordered by contacting Hay House (see next page).

***

We hope you enjoyed this Hay House book. If you'd like to receive our online catalog featuring additional information on Hay House books and products, or if you'd like to find out more about the Hay Foundation, please contact:

Hay House LLC, P.O. Box 5100, Carlsbad, CA 92018-5100
(760) 431-7695 or (800) 654-5126
www.hayhouse.com® • www.hayfoundation.org

———

Published in Australia by:
Hay House Australia Publishing Pty Ltd
18/36 Ralph St., Alexandria NSW 2015
Phone: +61 (02) 9669 4299
www.hayhouse.com.au

Published in the United Kingdom by:
Hay House UK Ltd
The Sixth Floor, Watson House,
54 Baker Street, London W1U 7BU
Phone: +44 (0) 203 927 7290
www.hayhouse.co.uk

Published in India by:
Hay House Publishers (India) Pvt Ltd
Muskaan Complex, Plot No. 3,
B-2, Vasant Kunj, New Delhi 110 070
Phone: +91 11 41761620
www.hayhouse.co.in

———

Let Your Soul Grow

Experience life-changing transformation—one video at a time—with guidance from the world's leading experts.

www.healyourlifeplus.com

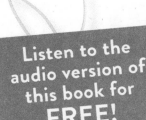
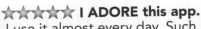

Free e-newsletters from Hay House, the Ultimate Resource for Inspiration

Be the first to know about Hay House's free downloads, special offers, giveaways, contests, and more!

 Get exclusive excerpts from our latest releases and videos from *Hay House Present Moments*.

 Our ***Digital Products Newsletter*** is the perfect way to stay up-to-date on our latest discounted eBooks, featured mobile apps, and Live Online and On Demand events.

 Learn with real benefits! *HayHouseU.com* is your source for the most innovative online courses from the world's leading personal growth experts. Be the first to know about new online courses and to receive exclusive discounts.

 Enjoy uplifting personal stories, how-to articles, and healing advice, along with videos and empowering quotes, within *Heal Your Life*.

Sign Up Now!

Get inspired, educate yourself, get a complimentary gift, and share the wisdom!

Visit www.hayhouse.com/newsletters to sign up today!